The battle against heart disease

T0292347

By the same author

The Battle against Bacteria

published by Cambridge University Press, 1965
translated into Norwegian, 1967; Japanese, 1968;
also Serbo-Croat, Czech and Hungarian in preparation.

P. E. BALDRY

M.B., B.S., M.R.C.P.
Fellow of the Royal
College of Physicians

The battle against heart disease

A physician traces the history of
man's achievements in this field
for the general reader

With a foreword by
J. F. GOODWIN M.D., F.R.C.P.
Professor of Clinical Cardiology
at Royal Postgraduate Medical School, London

CAMBRIDGE
at the University Press 1971

CAMBRIDGE UNIVERSITY PRESS
Cambridge, New York, Melbourne, Madrid, Cape Town, Singapore, São Paulo, Delhi

Cambridge University Press
The Edinburgh Building, Cambridge CB2 8RU, UK

Published in the United States of America by Cambridge University Press, New York

www.cambridge.org
Information on this title: www.cambridge.org/9780521103152

© Cambridge University Press 1971

First published 1971
This digitally printed version 2009

A catalogue record for this publication is available from the British Library

Library of Congress Catalogue Card Number: 75–108098

ISBN 978-0-521-07490-2 hardback
ISBN 978-0-521-10315-2 paperback

Foreword

THE rapid developments in the understanding of cardiovascular disorders add emphasis and drama to the continuously unfolding story of cardiology. Because of the increase in technology and the volume of publication it is often difficult to appreciate the background to, or the significance of, new developments. As the problems of cardiovascular disorders increase, so knowledge of the elements of heart disease becomes the more important for all readers. Thus it is a pleasure to read Dr Baldry's fascinating book which traces the history of heart disease from the sixth century B.C. to the present time. Dr Baldry writes clearly and concisely and has sifted a mass of historical material to put the essentials into a highly readable form, achieving a nice blend of historical anecdote with scientific detail.

Starting with early concepts of circulatory disease in the days of the Greek Empire, the text moves on through the Renaissance period, to the discovery of the circulation of the blood, early understanding of the structure and function of the heart, and finally to modern studies of hypertension, coronary artery disease and cardiac surgery.

Dr Baldry has a feeling for medical history that emerges clearly from his writing, and the characters who move through his pages have depth and reality. Despite the wealth of material the text is never dull. Both lay and medical readers should enjoy reading this book and profit from the opportunity to view recent advances against the backcloth of past discoveries.

September 1969   J. F. GOODWIN M.D., F.R.C.P.

To K.M.Y.

Contents

'Those who were before us did much, but they did not complete; much of the work yet still remains and much will remain, and the opportunity of adding something will not be denied to anyone born a thousand ages later.'

– SENECA

Preface

IN recent years much publicity has been given in the press and on television, to the efforts of the medical profession in their battle against heart disease. The purpose of this book is to give the general reader a better understanding of the subject by showing how our knowledge has gradually evolved.

It is also hoped that it will be of interest to doctors, medical students and nurses, because at a time when medicine is advancing so rapidly that textbooks are quickly out of date and what was taught fifty years ago appears strangely old-fashioned, there is an erroneous tendency to consider that the modern practice of medicine is based almost entirely on recent discoveries. This misapprehension can only be corrected by a study of history, when it becomes apparent that although there has been a rapid expansion of our knowledge in the present era, in conjunction with technological advances in science generally, medical practice is none the less still profoundly influenced by work of fundamental and lasting value contributed by many pioneers throughout the centuries.

My sincere thanks are due to Miss Kathleen Young for her interest, encouragement and untiring assistance in the preparation of the typescript for publication. Also, to Mr S. H. Watkins of the Wellcome Institute of the History of Medicine, whose knowledge and enthusiasm was of considerable help in my search for suitable illustrations.

P. E. B.

Acknowledgements

I gratefully acknowledge the permission to reproduce published illustrations granted by the holders of copyright, many of whom kindly supplied prints:

The *American Journal of Medical Sciences* for the electrocardiogram on p. 116; the Cambridge Instrument Company Ltd, Cambridge, for the photographs pp. 80 and 83 from S. L. Barron: *The development of the electrocardiograph*; Charing Cross Hospital Medical School and Longmans Group Ltd, for the figure p. 149; J. and A. Churchill Ltd, for the photograph of E. H. Starling, p. 40 from Starling: *Principles of human physiology*, 1941; Eyre and Spottiswoode for the figure p. 82 from Wood: *Diseases of the heart and circulation*; R. T. Gunther and Oxford University Press for the portrait of John Floyer, p. 86; Her Gracious Majesty the Queen for the drawing p. 11; the *Irish Journal of Medical Science* for the portrait of Robert Adams, p. 88; Mr John Jackson, F.R.C.S., of Harefield Hospital, Middlesex for the photographs on pp. 92 and 176; Dr Keith Jefferson of St George's Hospital and the National Heart Hospital for those on p. 180; National Library of Medicine for the portraits pp. 113 and 114; J. Playfair McMurrich for the self-portrait of Leonardo da Vinci, p. 9; Mrs Joan Prince and the Lister Institute of Preventive Medicine for the photograph of Sir Henry Dale, p. 40; *Punch* for the cartoon p. 135; and the Wellcome Institute Trustees for illustrations pp. 5, 6, 12, 13, 17, 20, 21, 24, 25, 27, 28, 38, 42, 43, 44, 49, 52, 54, 56, 58, 61, 64, 65, 68, 70, 71, 76, 77, 81, 83, 87, 89, 94, 95, 96, 107, 110, 112, 125, 137, 141, 142, 147. Diagrams on pp. 32, 160, 163, 164 are based on illustrations in *Congenital heart abnormalities*, Ross Laboratories; p. 36 is based on a diagram in C. Best and N. Taylor, *The physiological basis of medical practice*, Williams & Wilkins, 1945; p. 45 on a drawing in H. Dible & T. Davie, *Pathology*, Churchill, 1939; p. 178 is based on an illustration in an article by D. B. Effler in *Clinical Symposia* vol. 21, no. 1 1969.

P. E. B.

1

Preliminary reconnaissance by the early Greeks

THE evolution of knowledge of the heart and its function may be traced from manuscripts written in the early days of the Greek Empire several hundred years before Christ. Documents from earlier periods are few and inaccurate, although it is certain that the highly developed civilisations in Egypt and Mesopotamia possessed much scientific knowledge which had an important influence on Greek thought. The Ionians were the first Greeks to show an interest in science; they lived about 600 B.C. along the eastern shores of the Aegean Sea in an area bounded by Ephesus in the north and Hali-carnassus in the south. Their study of this began when Thales (*c.* 640–546 B.C.), a merchant who lived in the important city of

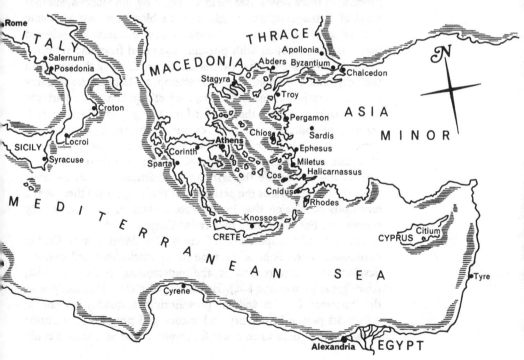

Map of the Ancient World showing some of the early centres of medicine and science

Miletus, learned about mathematics during his frequent business journeys to Egypt and Mesopotamia. Thales's application of this knowledge to practical problems in his home city led Anaximander (611–547 B.C.) with whom he studied mathematics to use these methods to calculate the size of the heavenly bodies and the distance between them. Anaximenes, born about 570 B.C., inspired by Anaximander's study of the cosmos, began to think about the properties of air, which he called pneuma. Pneuma, which literally means breath, or spirit, he considered to be the substance of the soul and the essence of life. It was soon recognised that this mysterious substance, permeating everywhere and everything, was drawn into the body by the rhythmic movements of the lungs and that its distribution around the body depended on a system of vessels. These vessels were first demonstrated about 500 B.C. by Alcmaeon, a pupil of Pythagoras, in Croton, a city in southern Italy, which was in the area then known as Magna Graeca. Pythagoras's pupils studied not only mathematics but biology and, making use of their remarkable artistic ability, produced intricate and detailed drawings of the external characteristics of animals. Alcmaeon went further than this, as he was the first to practise the scientific dissection of animals, and described the nerves linking the eyes to the brain, as well as the blood-containing vessels which ramify throughout the body. The function of these vessels was further studied by Empedocles, another pupil of Pythagoras, who taught that the blood contains an innate heat essential to life, closely associated with pneuma. He believed that this heat, together with pneuma, emanated from and returned to the heart, by moving backwards and forwards along the vessels in tidal rhythmic pulsations. The first attempt to describe the anatomy of these vessels was made by Diogenes of Apollonia in about 400 B.C.; he considered that they radiated from large vertical trunks and, because of differences in their external appearance, decided that there must be two types of vessel with separate functions. The early biologists soon discovered that some vessels in a dead animal are empty: this is because the last few contractions of a dying heart drive the blood towards the periphery of the body; it led them to the erroneous conclusion that in life also, certain of the vessels only contain air. For this reason they called them arteries.

The scientific importance of cities like Miletus and Croton diminished when Athens, because of its intellectual and cultural development, attracted to it the outstanding Ionian scientist, Anaxagoras (c. 500–430 B.C.). He developed a close friendship with the statesman Pericles and the poet Euripides, quickly became an influential person in the city and encouraged progress in scientific knowledge at a time when it was first realised that no one man could compass the whole of knowledge and that it was essential for individuals to specialise. The first two specialist schools in Athens were in medicine and mathematics and, by an extraordinary coincidence, their two leaders had the same name and came from neighbouring islands. They were the physician Hippocrates of Cos and the mathematician Hippocrates of Chios. Hippocrates the physician, born about 460 B.C., developed an outstanding system of medical practice, in which he not only formulated wise principles for the individual care of the patient but also initiated a method of observation from which stemmed many of the great advances in medicine. The accurate deductions of many of his followers were recorded in documents which are still available for our study and in one such treatise the concept that the blood vessels must link together to form a continuous circuit is clearly stated...

the vessels communicate with one another and the blood flows from one to another, I do not know where the commencement is to be found, for in a circle you can find neither commencement nor end, but from the heart the arteries take their origin and through the vessels the blood is distributed to all the body ... the heart and the vessels are perpetually moving, and we may compare the movement of the blood with courses of rivers returning to their sources after a passage through numerous channels.

It was another two thousand years before William Harvey was able to prove the veracity of this statement.

A document which was even more remarkable for its amazing clarity and accuracy, written by another member of the Hippocratic school and entitled 'On the Heart', describes the heart as a powerful muscle with two distinct ventricles, and observes that the beat of the left ventricle may be felt behind the left nipple. Also, it describes the auricles and gives a detailed description of the structure and function of the valves placed between these chambers. Some authorities consider that this manuscript was written about 340 B.C. by Philistion, a contemporary of Plato, but others think it must have been by another student of Hippocrates and written at a much later period. Although the author obviously had much knowledge of the structure of the heart, he was confused about its function, believing that it was the centre of the intellect and that air in the left ventricle was changed into a special type of pneuma or spirit before being distributed throughout the body; this idea was to persist with even greater elaboration up to the Middle Ages. The studies of the early Greeks were impeded by their not being allowed to dissect human bodies; Aristotle (384–322 B.C.) left wonderful accounts of the structure and function of the organs of many animals, but had an imperfect knowledge of the anatomy of the human heart, believing that it only had three chambers. However, one of his pupils, Praxagoras, who became an important medical teacher in the latter part of the third century B.C., made a detailed study of the pulsation felt in arteries, clearly distinguished arteries from veins, but persisted in the idea that the arteries contain air and that it is only the veins which contain blood.

When the importance of Athens as a city of culture diminished, the centre for scientific advance for many centuries was Alexandria. There, the study of anatomy advanced rapidly as dissection of the human body was now allowed. This change of attitude came about because the immigrant Greeks in Alexandria, who were far away from the superstitions and taboos of their native land, increasingly came to accept Plato's philosophy that the human body is no more than an expendable container in which the eternal soul temporarily resides. The first two Greek anatomists to take advantage of this new outlook were Herophilus and Erasistratus. Herophilus, about 300 B.C., developed a remarkably clear understanding of the workings of the heart and blood vessels and appreciated that although arteries are empty after death they contain blood during life, and made a detailed study of the rhythm and rate of the arterial pulse with the assistance of the clepsydra, a Greek instrument for measuring time by the regulated flow of water. Also he gave a most lucid account of the body's use of air, dividing the process into four distinct phases: the absorption of fresh air; its distribution in the body; its return to the lungs; and the exhalation of used air into the atmosphere. Such insight into the complex mechanism of the use of air by the body at that period was tantamount to genius. Erasistratus, his assistant, unfortunately supported the belief that the arteries only contain air. Although he knew that blood spurts from an injured artery, he explained this by saying that the blood must have come from a vein and have been drawn into the vacuum produced by the air escaping from the damaged artery. This ingenious hypothesis, though erroneous, led him to the correct conclusion that the arteries and veins must be connected by a network of minute vessels or capillaries. It was not, of course, until the invention of the microscope, centuries later, that these vessels could be seen. Erasistratus understood that the heart valves ensure unidirectional flow of blood but was prevented from a complete understanding of the circulation by his support of the theory that arteries contain air.

The writings of Herophilus and Erasistratus were lost in the great fire which destroyed the library at Alexandria so that our knowledge of these two men is based on accounts given to us by Galen four centuries later. Galen (A.D. c. 130–200), after completing his study of medicine at Alexandria, returned to his native town of Pergamon in Asia Minor, to take charge of the gladiators, an appointment which must have given him much experience in the treatment of wounds.

In the year 162 he moved to Rome where he soon became well known for his skill in the performance of experiments and dissection of animals, whilst at the same time he was greatly respected as a practising physician. His diagnostic acumen from observations of the pulse is well illustrated by an account of his management of two patients. On being called to examine a young woman he noted that she had no fever and a normal pulse rate, except when the name of a certain actor was mentioned, when it increased in speed and became irregular. On two subsequent visits, therefore, he purposely spoke about another actor and observed that this did not affect her pulse, so on the fourth occasion he again mentioned the name of the first actor and from the fact that her pulse rate immediately increased concluded that her illness was of emotional origin and stemmed from unrequited love! The second occasion was when three physicians who, from an examination of the Emperor, Marcus Aurelius, considered he was sickening for a fever, but Galen, from a close observation of the character of his pulse, correctly diagnosed that the Emperor was suffering from no more than a distended stomach from overeating!

Dissection of the human body had once again been forbidden so that all Galen's observations had to be made on animals. He not only dissected but also vivisected many farm animals such as sheep, horses and cows, as well as wild animals, including lynxes, bears, lions and at least one elephant, in addition to birds, fish and snakes. He was a most skilful operator and his enquiring mind led him to conduct most ingenious and carefully contrived experiments to see what happened when muscles were cut, nerves severed, or various tubes and ducts ligated in live animals. From his experiments he learned about the control of respiration and phonation by nerves from the spinal cord, and from ligation of various parts of the urinary tract demonstrated the function of the kidneys. Much of his study

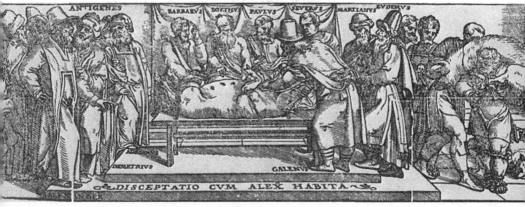

Galen (c. A.D. 130–200) vivisecting a pig

of the heart's action was done on the exposed, beating hearts of pigs and sheep. It took him some time to develop a satisfactory technique of opening the chest so that initially many of his animals died but with experience he became more successful and in *On Anatomical Procedures* he wrote, '...when the heart is exposed, your task is to preserve all its functions unimpaired, as in fact they are, so that you can see the animal breathing and uttering cries and, if loosed from its bonds, running as before...'. Unfortunately, a pig's heart beats so quickly that he had much difficulty in analysing the movements of its various chambers and the direction in which the blood flowed through them. When dissecting snakes he did not take advantage of examining their slower acting hearts, as did William Harvey fifteen hundred years later. Although Galen came to certain valid conclusions about the heart's action he also made many grave errors. He

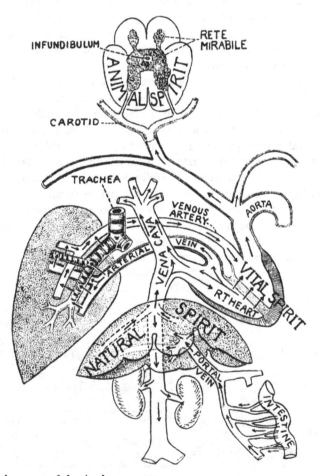

Galen's concept of the circulatory system

realised, unlike his predecessors, that arteries, as well as veins, contained blood, he had a good understanding that the action of the valves was to ensure unidirectional blood flow, but his teaching was not consistent in this matter for when it suited his purpose he postulated that there could be two streams flowing in opposite directions.

His explanation of the movement of blood was most complex. He taught that chyle from the intestine flowed into the liver, where it was transformed into blood which became imbued at that site with a special type of pneuma called natural spirit; charged with this, the blood was then distributed by the veins to the body. Some of the blood, flowing through one of the larger veins called the vena cava, reached the right ventricle where some, but not all, was directed into what he called 'the artery-like vein' (the pulmonary artery) to reach the lungs; blood from the lungs travelled along what he called 'the vein-like artery' (pulmonary vein) to return to the left ventricle. He somewhat confusingly ascribed three other functions to this vessel, believing that the air inhaled into the lungs from the atmosphere travelled in a separate stream alongside the blood and that it was not until the left ventricle was reached that the blood mixed with the air, with the production of vital spirit. He considered that while most of this spiritous blood was distributed by the aorta to the body a small part of it flowed in the opposite direction along the 'vein-like artery' in order to nourish the lungs and that this stream of blood was accompanied by a separate outflow of waste material which escaped to the atmosphere via the lungs. Although this explanation appears muddled and cumbersome to us, Galen must be given credit for his understanding that waste material is expelled from the lungs, at the same time that fresh air is absorbed. A major error, and one that led him into much confusion, was his belief that the interaction of air and blood takes place in the left ventricle rather than in the lungs. But his biggest mistake was his belief that part of the blood in the right ventricle reached the left ventricle by percolating through invisible pores in the septum separating these two chambers.

Galen expressed his views with strong conviction and it might appear that he inherited the intellect of his father and the domineering character of his mother because, he tells us, '...my father was amiable, just and benevolent, my mother on the other hand had a very bad temper, she used to bite her serving maids and was perpetually shouting at my father'. His teachings, though inaccurate, were accepted as gospel not only during his own life but until the Renaissance.

2

Reappraisal during the Renaissance

PROGRESS in medical science in the Graeco-Roman civilisation ended with the achievements of Galen. His belief that his teaching of anatomy was an accurate account of the design of nature as created by God was accepted by Christian, Moslem and Jewish theologians who conferred on his writings a spiritual blessing and religious approbation which made any attempt at contradiction blasphemous and heretical. This attitude naturally removed any further desire for investigation or enquiry and was to bring scientific progress to a halt for a thousand years.

After the fall of the Roman Empire, the Christian Church discouraged orthodox medicine because, although Christ healed the sick, his followers considered that disease was inflicted as a punishment for sin which was only to be expiated by prayer and repentance. This suppressive attitude affected not only medicine but science in general and reached its climax in A.D. 391 when a mob of fanatics set fire to the great library at Alexandria, destroying many priceless treasures of ancient science. Intellectual leadership passed in about the eighth century to people of Arabic speech, including not only the citizens of Arabia but also some Syrians, Persians and Spaniards, whose appreciation of the importance of Greek medicine was far more enlightened. Their physicians, not all Moslems, some Christians, others Jews, were united in their desire to spread the knowledge of medicine and for this purpose translated the works of their Greek predecessors into Arabic. A very influential Arabic scientist and writer in the tenth century was Rhazes, whose greatest medical work *The Comprehensive Book* was one of the most extensive ever written and included virtually the whole of Greek, Syrian and Arabic medical knowledge. A century later another outstanding Moslem, Ibn Sina, known to the Western world as Avicenna, integrated Greek and Moslem medical knowledge in his famous *Canon* in which he reiterated Galen's views, including his description of the heart and lungs. The first person to question Galen's authority

was the Arab physician Ibn Nafis who, about the middle of the
thirteenth century in his *Commentary on the Anatomy of Avicenna's
Canon*, rejected the assumption made by Galen and perpetuated by
Avicenna, that there are pores in the interventricular septum through
which blood passes from the right ventricle to mix with air in the
left ventricle, and expressed his belief that the aeration of blood takes
place in the lungs. Such a concept was centuries ahead of its time
and because of this was ignored, being unacceptable in the prevailing
climate of opinion. Nothing more was heard of this commentary
until translated into Latin by Andreas Alpagos and his nephew on
their return to Padua in 1520, after spending many years in the East.
Recently, Arab authorities have claimed that it was this translation
that brought about the anti-Galenic movement in Padua in the
sixteenth century but, unfortunately, the anatomical section of their
translation cannot be found so that it is not possible to judge the
extent of its influence. The original manuscript was rediscovered by
an Egyptian medical student Muhyi el din At Tatawi in the archives
of the Prussian State Library in 1922. Part of it was then published
by him in a university thesis in 1924 and thirty-one years later the
entire work was translated into English by E. Bittar, a graduate of
Yale Medical School.

The revolt against the unquestioning acceptance of Galen's
authoritative teaching coincided with man's determination to escape
from the unswerving, narrow, tyrannical attitudes of the Church and
the dry, unthinking dogmatism of scholars. This renaissance, as is
well known, began about the end of the fourteenth century in
Florence and gradually spread across Europe to reach England in the
Elizabethan era. This movement, which liberated thoughts and
attitudes, led to a reappraisal of science, literature and art. One
important change was that the beauty of the human form could now
be admired without feelings of guilt or shame, so that artists felt
inspired and encouraged to portray its true likeness, but as anatomists,
still blinded by prejudice, could not teach them, they had to turn to
dissection themselves. Michelangelo, Raphael, and Albrecht Dürer
were amongst the great artists who studied in detail the bone structure and contours of the superficial muscles but the most outstanding
was Leonardo da Vinci (1452–1519) who, not content with this,
dissected the deeper structures of the body. His original, enquiring
mind led him to be a brilliant inventor as well as a great anatomist
and artist. His knowledge ranged over all branches of science from
mathematics to physiology, though often his grasp of principles was
far ahead of the time when they could be of practical use. Thus he
designed a parabolic compass and made drawings of quick-firing and
breech-loading guns long before technical skill permitted their

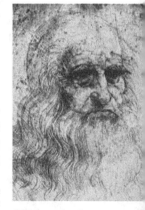

*Self-portrait of
Leonardo da Vinci
(1452–1519)*

manufacture. His study of flight in birds led him to devise a model
of a flying machine and to plan the construction of a helicopter and
parachute. As engineer in charge of the maintenance of the water-
ways in Lombardy, he studied the mechanical principles underlying
the movement of water in rivers and streams by making model glass
channels and observing the flow of water with the help of added
millet seeds, fragments of papyrus and seeds of panic grass '... so
that one can see the course of the water better from their movements'.
It was these same methods which he was to use in later years when
he came to study the action of the heart.

Contrary to Galen's belief, Leonardo was quick to realise that the
heart is made of muscle which acts as a pump so that blood which
flows into it in its relaxed state (diastole) is forced out under pressure
when it contracts (systole). His great interest in hydrodynamics and
his genius for invention led him to devise working models whereby
he could simulate the action of this pump and study in particular the
movement of the valves, without having to resort to vivisection, a
practice which he strongly abhorred. It was the valve at the mouth
of the aorta which he studied most intensively and he showed that
when a stream of blood enters the aorta from the left ventricle the
valve shuts immediately to prevent the blood regurgitating. This is
now relatively easy to demonstrate by ciné-radiography after the
injection of radio-opaque dyes into the circulation, but for Leonardo
it was a task which demanded consummate skill and ingenuity.
First he made a solid cast of the aorta by pouring wax into it from
above and allowing it to flow through the valve opening into the
heart. From this he prepared a hollow cast of gypsum which he lined
with a sheet of blown glass. Then he fashioned a cast of the valve
which he incorporated into this glass mould in order, he said, 'to see
in the glass what the blood does in the heart when it shuts the
opening of the valves'. Both from his observations of dissection
specimens and study of his cast, he learned that the aorta is of
triangular shape and that its mouth where the valve cusps are
inserted is widened by three flanges, later to be known as the
sinuses of Valsalva. With his glass model and the use of grass seed
he performed experiments from which he deduced that when blood
is ejected into the aorta turbulence is set up so that, in addition to
the main jet, there are three vortices which by a backward sweep
into the sinuses of Valsalva close the valve cusps by sideways pressure.
He went to much trouble to demonstrate this phenomenon in his
drawings and to point out that the valve cusps could not be closed
by simple vertical pressure from the weight of the main stream of
blood above them as this would cause them to buckle. It is incredible
that Leonardo learned all this from the movement of grass seed in a

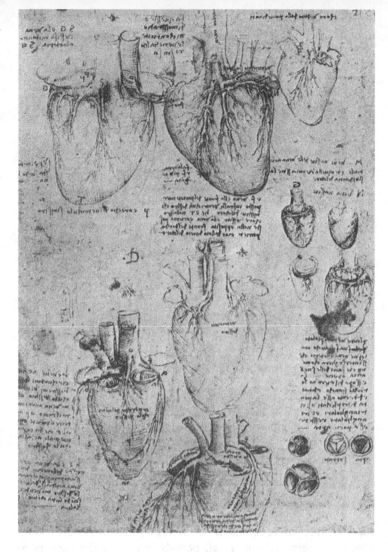

Drawings of the heart and coronary vessels by Leonardo da Vinci

glass tube, especially as recent attempts to repeat similar experiments have not been successful.

He has left many beautiful drawings of his models and of the valves as seen both in the closed and open positions. He must have seen them in motion as he drew the cusps with a wrinkled edge, an appearance not seen in the closed valve after death. He placed his illustrations in order across the page from right to left as he was left-handed and always wrote in that direction. Most of his drawings have very little explanatory text so that often his meaning is expressed entirely by pictorial sequence, as his power of literary expression was limited. His sentences, often ungrammatical, frequently unfinished, were at times monotonously repetitive as he tried to emphasise his meaning by writing passages two or three times. He was much aware of his difficulties in writing but maintained that visual images are

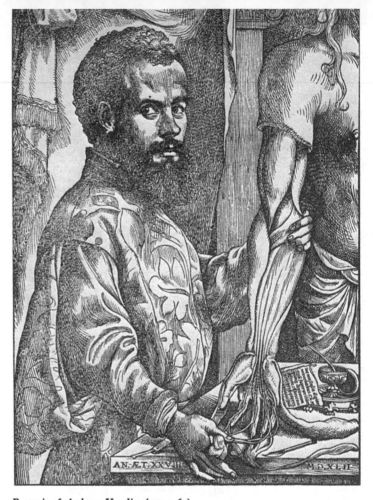

Portrait of Andreas Vesalius (1514–64)

superior in scientific communications as they may be understood by people of every language in all periods and avoid the dangers of translation errors. Certainly, once his method of visual expression is understood it is easy to follow his meaning and his paucity of descriptive words does not detract from the importance of his scientific achievements. His anatomical and physiological studies were not surpassed in many respects for several centuries but regrettably the vast compilation of notes and drawings which he hoped to assemble in the last years of his life was never published. Bequeathed to a friend, they gradually became divided and scattered in successive generations having little influence on the advancement of science and being of value to few except modern historians.

The revision of anatomical knowledge initiated by artists was continued by Andreas Vesalius (1514–64) the first anatomist to base his teaching of the subject on personal observations of the structure of the human body instead of blindly following Galen's dogma. Born in Brussels he learned anatomy first at Louvain and then in Paris: his teachers, Jacobus Sylvius and Johannes Günther, were ardent Galenists, Sylvius being so bigoted that when he found any structure not conforming to Galen's description he argued that it must be because of degeneration of the human species since Galen's time. It is not surprising that he strongly disapproved of Vesalius, whereas Günther encouraged the development of his pupil's lively mind. Vesalius realised early in his student life that to learn anatomy accurately he would have to dissect the human body himself. As this was not part of the university curriculum the authorities made no arrangements for a regular supply of bodies so that Vesalius himself, often at great personal risk, had to visit gibbets, cemeteries and charnel-houses in the course of various body-snatching escapades. His enthusiastic expenditure of so much energy had its reward when in 1536 at Louvain, one year before qualification, he had the honour of conducting the first public dissection to be held there for many years.

He received his doctorate of medicine on 5 December 1537 and almost immediately was appointed Professor of Surgery and Anatomy at the University of Padua. It was the usual custom in those days for a professor of anatomy to expound Galenic theories seated in his academic chair but Vesalius taught from personally conducted dissections. As he realised that much of the traditional teaching was

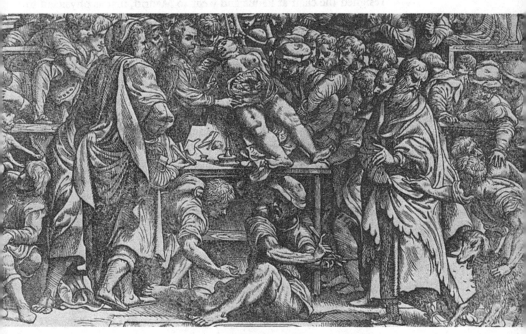

An anatomy lesson by Vesalius

wrong he often found himself in angry clashes with his contemporaries but his students, recognising his merits, came in large numbers to his classes. At the early age of twenty-eight he published his book *De Humani Corporis Fabrica* which contains most beautiful drawings, executed with great artistic skill. The illustrations of the muscles of the body are superb and admirably portray their appearances in action as well as at rest. This was done because he recognised the importance of learning not only about the structure of an organ but also of studying the mechanism by which it worked. Like Leonardo he made a special study of the heart and, in the first edition of his book, supported Galen's teaching about invisible septal pores though it is obvious that this concept worried him because he wrote, '... we are compelled to wonder at the industry of the Creator of all things by which the blood sweats from the right ventricle into the left ventricle through invisible pores...!' In the second edition he was no longer able to support this view for he said, 'I have not found even the most hidden passages ... not long ago I would not have dared to turn aside, even a nail's breadth, from the opinion of Galen, the prince of physicians ... but the septum of the heart is as thick, dense and compact, as the rest of the heart'.

Once this treatise on anatomy had been published his career as a teacher unfortunately ended. He had revolutionised anatomy but in so doing had made many enemies. Possibly because of this he resigned the chair at Padua and went to Madrid, first as physician to the Emperor Charles V and later to his son Philip II. Little is known of his life in Spain except that in 1564 he left Madrid on a pilgrimage to Jerusalem: it appears that while performing a post-mortem examination on a Spanish nobleman the seeming corpse suddenly showed signs of life. The Church dignitaries considered that this startling event was evidence that he had committed the heinous crime of vivisection, pardonable only by a visit of repentance to the Holy Land. As this was the time of the Inquisition, Vesalius had no alternative but to comply with their demand. On the return journey his ship was wrecked near the Gulf of Corinth and there, in October 1564, he died. His career as an anatomist was brief but his contributions to the subject were so profound as to supplant those of Galen. From this time it was Vesalian anatomy which was generally taught and it was at Padua that William Harvey studied anatomy thirty-three years later.

Vesalius's assistant, Realdus Columbus (1516–80), who succeeded him as Professor of Anatomy, continued his work on the heart concluding that the blood in the right ventricle reaches the left ventricle by passing through the lungs. In his *De Re Anatomica* in 1559 he said, 'this fact no one has hitherto observed or recorded in writing: yet it may most readily be observed by anyone'. This was not correct because, unknown to him, Michael Servetus had been burnt at the stake six years earlier for publishing a similar view.

Michael Servetus was primarily a theologian and devout Christian whose only crime was his unwillingness to accept blindly the doctrine of the Church. As a young man, from his studies of the Greek and Hebrew Bibles, he found he was unable to support the theory of the Trinity and had the courage to say so, publishing his views at the age of twenty, whilst at the same time prudently changing his name to Villanovanus.

After completing his medical studies in Paris he worked as a doctor in the small French town of Vienne where, in addition to his routine practice, he spent much time in medical and theological research. Although he changed his name he seemed determined to court disaster by communicating his religious views to Calvin. Not content with this, in 1553 he published anonymously his extensive work *Christianismi Restitutio*. This book, for the most part concerned with theology, also included his contributions to physiology because he considered that the two were inextricably linked. He described the change in colour that takes place in blood when it mixes with air in the lungs and particularly emphasised that the pulmonary artery, because of its large size, must have a more important function than that of just transporting blood to the lungs for their nourishment, whilst at the same time expressing disbelief in Galen's septal pores. Unfortunately for Servetus he was identified as the author by a friend of Calvin and arrested. He escaped from prison and went to Geneva, but whilst attending a church service there one Sunday morning was recognised, immediately put on trial by the Magistracy, and on 27 October 1553, burnt at the stake with a copy of the offending book placed under his arm. He lost his life because of his departure from Galenic orthodoxy but may not have considered the price too much for at the close of his book he wrote, 'he who really understands what is involved in the breathing of man, has already sensed the breath of God and thereby saved his soul'.

3

The circulation discovered

THE first Englishman to make a notable contribution to our understanding of the heart's action was William Harvey, born in Folkestone on 1 April 1578. His education at the King's School, Canterbury started in the year of the defeat of the Spanish Armada. He became very proficient in Latin and Greek and later in life evidently thought in Latin as many of his scientific notes were written in a curious mixture of Latin and English. At the age of sixteen he went to Gonville and Caius College, Cambridge, with a scholarship of £3 8d. per annum to continue his classical education. About this time Dr Caius, one of the founders of the College, who had a particular interest in anatomy, obtained permission for the bodies of two criminals to be dissected at his College each year, but it is not definitely known whether Harvey, as a Classics scholar, was allowed to watch. Having obtained his Bachelor of Arts degree in 1597, he went to the University of Padua to study medicine because of its great reputation for teaching anatomy since the time of Vesalius. The Professor of Anatomy in his time was Hieronymus Fabricius who, in 1594, at his own expense, had built a new anatomy amphitheatre at the University. Fabricius was obviously a great inspiration to Harvey for later in his life in his book *De motu cordis* he refers with great affection to his former teacher.

While Harvey was at Padua, Fabricius made a special study of the valves, along the course of veins. These he called ostiola or little doors but misunderstood their proper function, thinking that they were to prevent the over distension of veins by a backward flow of blood and failed to appreciate that their main function, conversely, is to assist the forward passage of blood up veins towards the heart. Harvey told Robert Boyle, the famous physicist, that it was Fabricius's interest in these valves when he was a student that led him later to re-examine them for himself and, by a study of their position and structure, obtained much help in his understanding of the circulation of the blood.

After five years at Padua, Harvey passed his final examination with distinction and on his return to England also obtained his doctorate of medicine from the University of Cambridge. In 1609, at the age of thirty-one, he became a physician on the teaching staff of St Bartholomew's Hospital, London, and six years later was honoured by being appointed the Lumleian lecturer to the Royal College of Physicians. It is extremely fortunate that the manuscript notes referring to the second day's lecture on 17 April 1616, by some extraordinary chance, found their way into the British Museum where they were discovered in 1886, some two hundred and seventy years later. They are of particular importance as there, for the first time, the fact that the blood circulates round the body was clearly and unequivocally stated. Harvey wrote:

It is plain, from the structure of the heart, that the blood is passed continuously through the lungs to the aorta as by two clacks of a water-bellows to raise water. It is shown, by application of a ligature, that the passage of blood is from the arteries into the veins. Whence it follows that the movement of the blood is constantly in a circle and is brought about by the beat of the heart....

His analogy of the heart to a pump is interesting, as a one-way valve instrument for drawing water out of mines had been invented in the late fifteenth and early sixteenth century and by Harvey's time must have been in common use. Although it is obvious, from these lecture notes, that Harvey recognised that blood circulates round the body, it was another twelve years before, in 1628, he published *Exercitatio anatomica de motu cordis et sanguinis in animalibus. De*

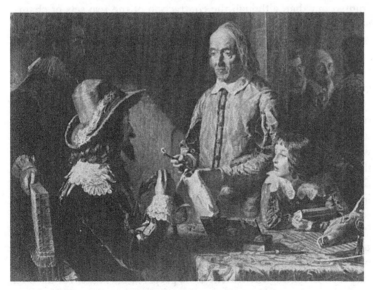

Harvey demonstrating the discovery of the circulation of the blood to Charles I

motu cordis, as it is often called, although only a small volume of seventy-four pages, was of the greatest importance, as it not only established the truth about the circulation of blood but it also described experimental methods devised by Harvey which were to form the basis for all future work in physiology.

When Harvey first tried to examine the heart's action he was thwarted, as others had been before him, by the speed of its movement. One of his first steps to solve this difficulty was to examine its action in cold-blooded animals, such as frogs, snakes and small fish. As vivisection interferes with the movement of the heart, with much ingenuity he studied animals, such as shrimps, whose transparent walls allowed the heart's action to be directly observed. It was from such studies, as well as from his post-mortem examination of human beings, that he formulated conclusions which he recorded logically and systematically in his book. He emphasised that the blood is expelled from the heart with each contraction and flows into it with each relaxation, an obvious fact now but one which had hitherto been the subject of much contention. Also he gives evidence to show that the contraction of the heart muscle coincides with expansion of the arteries which are then filled by a positive pressure transmitted from the heart, contrary to the opinion held up to that time that arteries expand like bellows and suck blood into them by a negative pressure. Also until then it was generally taught that each of the auricles and each of the ventricles contract independently, and Harvey was the first to show that both auricles contract together and that this is followed by simultaneous contraction of the two ventricles. He pointed out that, although the contraction of the two sets of chambers are distinct, they occur so rapidly as to appear to coincide, in the same way as the separate movements of the different parts of a gun appear to be one when fired. Further, in spite of the clear teaching of Vesalius which rejected much of Galen's views, Harvey still paid great deference to the Greek physician and was not willing to discount his views without the most careful presentation of closely reasoned arguments. His dissection studies enabled him to agree with Vesalius that the septum between the ventricles is solid, and with Columbus that all the blood from the right ventricle passes through the lungs to the left ventricle. He was unaware that Michael Servetus had come to the same conclusion because the three surviving copies of *Christianismi Restitutio* were not discovered for another seventy years. Harvey accepted Galen's belief that the action of the valves is to ensure unidirectional flow of blood but made no reference to the work of Leonardo da Vinci on this subject, since his writings were not available to him. As the book progresses one can sense Harvey's mounting excitement as he prepares the reader for his final conclusions by exclaiming:

But what remains to be said upon the quantity and source of the blood which thus passes, is of so novel and unheard of character, that I not only fear injury to myself from the envy of a few, but I tremble lest I have mankind at large for my enemies, so much doth wont and custom, that become as another nature, and doctrine once sown and that has struck deep root, and respect for antiquity influences all men. Still the die is cast, and my trust is in my love of truth, and the candour that inheres in cultivated minds.

This passage is quoted at length because it vividly portrays Harvey's realisation that his overthrow of long accepted teachings might lead to acrimony and possibly physical violence from his contemporaries. Undeterred however by any such considerations he continues by saying that, when he reflected on the large size of the chambers of the heart and the wide calibre of the blood vessels, he realised that they must contain a large volume of blood whose rate of flow would quickly empty the veins and fill the arteries to bursting unless it found its way back from the arteries through the veins, or, as he says, with evident excitement, writing his words in capitals, 'I began to think whether there might not be A MOTION, AS IT WERE, IN A CIRCLE.' He supports this argument by astute calculations pointing out that, as the ventricle holds approximately 2 oz (60 ml), if the pulse beats 72 times in a minute then in one hour the left ventricle drives into the aorta 540 lb (245 kg) of blood—three times the weight of a heavy man! Harvey asks where can all this blood have come from unless it passes round the body time and again in a circle. Finally, he describes his experiments with skilfully applied ligatures which enabled him to elucidate the direction of flow in arteries and veins, and gives his reappraisal of the function of the valves in the veins.

Harvey did not suffer physical injury when his book was published but had to face much scorn and derision which temporarily damaged his reputation and standing as one of the foremost physicians. As Physician to the royal household, Harvey often had to accompany the King or members of his Court on official journeys and it must therefore have been with a certain amount of relief that he could escape from the hostile atmosphere of London when ordered by Charles I to accompany the Duke of Lennox on a journey to France and Spain. He always took every opportunity when travelling to find something of scientific interest to study, although on that particular occasion it appears that he was unlucky as he wrote to Lord Dorchester, Secretary of State, complaining that he could scarce see a dog, cow, kite or any other bird or other thing, to anatomise. He must have been more fortunate when he accompanied the Earl of Arundel to Germany because he was then so busy observing unusual

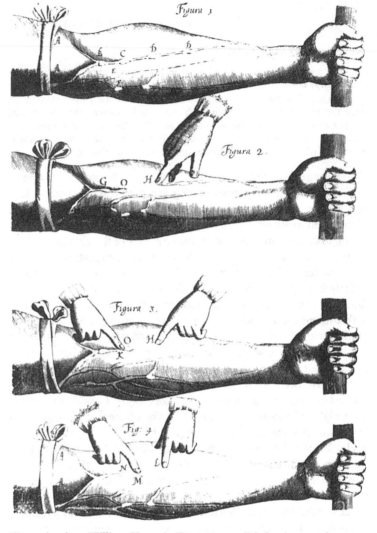

Illustration from William Harvey's 'De motu cordis' showing experiments to demonstrate the function of the valves of the vein

trees and plants that he incurred the Ambassador's displeasure by losing his way. In 1633, when he had the honour to accompany Charles I on his historic journey to Scotland for his coronation at Holyrood, Harvey found time to visit Edinburgh where he studied the wild life on the Bass Rock and in particular the habits of the gannets, or solan geese, which congregate there in large numbers.

As Royal Physician Harvey often had to give his expert opinion in unusual circumstances. In 1634, when seven Leicester women were accused of witchcraft because they were considered responsible for a storm which endangered the King's life on his voyage to Holyrood, Harvey, together with Alexander Baker and William Clowes, surgeons to the King, and six other medical men and ten midwives, had to examine these unfortunate women at The Ship Tavern in Greenwich. Their report stated that they had not found any stigmata of witchcraft on these women's bodies, including no evidence of satanic branding or diabolical intercourse; in spite of this only four of the women were pardoned. Shortly after this Harvey had to make another unusual examination when ordered by the King to perform an autopsy on the body of Thomas Parr, to find the reason for his long life as he was reported to have reached the age of one hundred and fifty-three at the time of his death. Parr spent most of his life in Shropshire, where he married twice, first at the age of eighty-eight and again when one hundred and twenty. Eventually he came to London in the service of the Earl of Arundel and it was there that he died. Harvey reported that his death was due to pleuro-pneumonia brought on by the impure air of London. This must have given scant comfort to the King particularly as he added that in his opinion the man would have lived even longer had he remained in rural Shropshire and avoided the rich diet of a nobleman's household.

Harvey obviously derived advantage from his close association with royalty but it also at times exposed him to danger. He was accused of having poisoned James I after attending him during his final illness and it was only after he had appeared before the House of Commons that he was exonerated. Because of his friendship with Charles I, his house was ransacked by a mob of soldiers during the Civil War and many of his important scientific papers were destroyed and goods looted. Also, when with the King's forces at Edgehill, his life was endangered by a stray cannon shot whilst reading a book to the King's two young sons near the battlefield.

Harvey was elected Warden of Merton College, Oxford, in 1645, but when that city surrendered to Cromwell in the same year he withdrew from public life. He presented to the Royal College of Physicians his large collection of books on science, natural history and travel, together with numerous other objects of interest including a variety of surgical instruments. An invitation, in 1654, to become President of the College, had to be regretfully declined as for some years his health had been seriously affected by recurrent attacks of gout. His affection for his College led him, in 1656, to donate to it his country estate at Burmash in Kent, on condition that the revenue should be used to provide an annual feast for the Fellows and an oration on the same day to commemorate benefactors and to exhort the Fellows to search and study out the secrets of nature by way of experiment. His death from a cerebral haemorrhage was on 3 June 1657, and he was buried in the family vault at Hempstead in Essex.

4

Respiration and its purpose

THE function of the lungs remained a mystery for many centuries; most of what Galen taught was confusing and inaccurate and although Harvey praised him for being the first man to describe the pulmonary circulation, he found that his ideas about it were unacceptable. Harvey too, in spite of his considerable knowledge of the circulation of blood, had much difficulty in understanding the purpose of the passage of the blood through the lungs. At first he said that it was so that the hot blood carried to and through the lungs could be tempered by the inspired air and freed from bubbling to excess. This obviously did not satisfy him and for the rest of his life the purpose of respiration exercised his mind. In his *Praelectiones* he remarks that there is no life without breathing and no breathing without life and wonders why it is that air is needed by animals which breathe just as it is required by a candle in order to burn. He promised to write a treatise on the subject but never progressed further than, just before his death, retracting his original traditional Galenic type of explanation and offering in its place the negative comment that air is given to animals neither for cooling nor as a nutrient. Chemistry had not sufficiently advanced for him to understand the properties of air and he was also handicapped by not being able to see how contact is made between the blood and air in the lungs, as the microscopes in use during his time were not sufficiently powerful.

The invention of the microscope stemmed from an understanding of the physical properties of mirrors and lenses first developed by Arabic physicists in the tenth century. Alhazen (965–1038), who was familiar with the laws of refraction and magnification, opposed the theory of Euclid and Ptolemy that the eye actively sends out rays in order to identify objects and stated in *The Treasury of Optics* that rays of light pass from the object to the eye and are there brought into focus by a lens. In Europe we are indebted to Robert Grosse-teste (*c.* 1175–1253) the Bishop of Lincoln who, after reading a Latin translation of Alhazen's works, carried out experiments with lenses himself and interested Roger Bacon (1214–94), amongst others, in the subject. Bacon was not only the first man to consider the possible use of lenses as spectacles but also, by his suggestion that lenses might be used in combination, was the progenitor of the microscope and telescope. The first microscope was invented about 1590 by Johann and Zacharias Janssen, two Dutch spectacle-makers

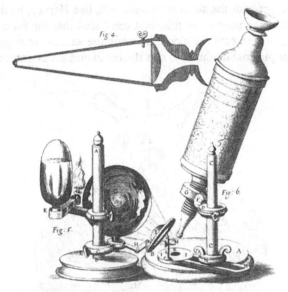

An early microscope used in the seventeenth century

in Middelburg. The power of this instrument was greatly increased towards the end of Harvey's life, when in 1646 Fontana modified the eye-piece, and enabled Malpighi, fourteen years later, to see the detailed structure of the lungs, including the capillaries linking the arteries and veins, as predicted already by Harvey.

Marcello Malpighi (1628–94) was born at Crevalcuore, near Bologna, and because of difficulties encountered in the settling of his family estate after the sudden death of his parents, did not start the study of medicine until the age of twenty-three, making up for lost time by only taking two years to qualify. One of Malpighi's professors, Bartolommeo Massari, frequently invited to his home some of the lecturers and more able students to discuss Harvey's work and conduct dissections. Malpighi found this experience of great benefit in laying the foundations for his future research at Pisa and Bologna. At Pisa, Malpighi became very friendly with Giovanni Borelli the mathematician and it was in two letters, written to him in 1660, that Malpighi first described the microscopic appearance of the lung

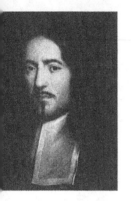

Portrait of Malpighi (1628–94)

structure. In the first letter he gave an account of the minute air-containing vesicles or alveoli at the termination of the bronchioles in the lungs of a dog, and in the second he described the flow of blood through the capillaries adjacent to the alveoli which he had so skilfully and cleverly seen on examination of the lungs of a living frog while the heart was still beating. He appreciated that the capillaries link the arteries and veins and that the blood in them comes into close contact with the air in the alveoli but, like Harvey, he did not understand the purpose of this. Not convinced that the function of the lungs was to cool the blood, he made the alternative suggestion that their purpose might be to mix the blood and act as a storehouse for it.

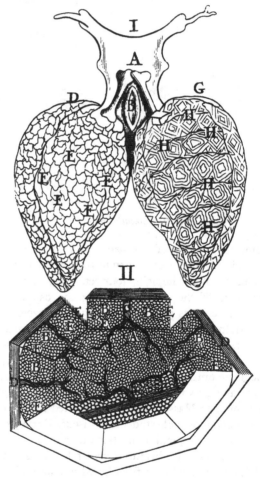

Malpighi's illustration of a microscopic section of the lung showing the alveolocapillary network

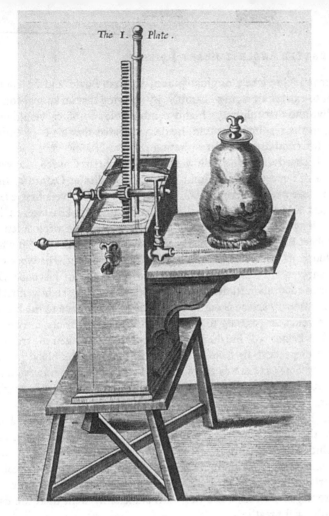

Boyle's air-pump used by him to produce a vacuum in a flask to demonstrate that air is essential for respiration

Malpighi's long life, during which he made many important anatomical discoveries, was marred towards its end when his house was burned down in 1684, destroying many of his microscopes and precious manuscripts, and also by vindictive attacks directed against him by his former close friend Borelli. His last three years were spent as personal physician to Pope Innocent XII in Rome, where he died in July 1694.

Understanding of the true purpose of respiration had to wait for another hundred and fifty years until physics and chemistry had become sufficiently advanced. The first man to make a scientific study of air was Robert Boyle (1627–91) who, with his pupil Robert Hooke at Oxford, made use of the air-pump invented in 1656 by Otto von Guericke (1602–86) Burgomaster of Magdeburg in Prussia. Hooke, who had great talent as an experimental physicist, considerably improved Guericke's original pump, so that Boyle and he could use it to extract air from a chamber. By showing that an animal could not live and that sulphur, a highly combustible substance, would not burn in the resultant vacuum, he demonstrated that air is essential both for combustion and respiration. Hooke became very friendly with Richard Lower, a fellow student at Christ Church. Lower, born at Tremeer, near Bodmin, began his studies at Oxford at the age of seventeen, where he soon proved himself to have a first-class intellect and to be highly skilled as an anatomist. His interest in physiology became evident when on 24 June 1664, he wrote a letter to Robert Boyle stating that he wished to investigate the reason why the blood in veins and arteries is of a different colour. His work on this subject, the results of which were published in his book *De Corde* in 1669, showed that blood withdrawn from the right ventricle and pulmonary artery is dark and similar in appearance to the blood in the veins, in contrast to blood from the left ventricle and aorta which is bright red. Further, he demonstrated that when the trachea is tied to prevent air from getting into the lungs, the blood in the aorta becomes as dark as that in the veins. From these observations he argued that the change in colour of the blood from dark to bright red must occur as a result of air mixing with the blood as it passes through the lungs and that the blood must revert to a dark red colour when the air it contains is absorbed by the tissues in the body. He concluded, 'from this it is easy to imagine the great advantage accruing to the blood from the admixture of air and the greater importance attaching to the air being always healthy and pure ... wherever, in a word, a fire can burn sufficiently well, there we can equally well breathe'.

Stephen Hales, a Teddington clergyman, with a remarkable ability for scientific investigation whose life will be discussed more fully in chapter 14 was the first man to measure quantitatively the amount of air used during respiration. In 1733, in his *Statical Essays* he described the ingenious but simple apparatus invented by him to measure the quantity of air absorbed during breathing, while at the same time he marvelled at the vast surface area of the alveolo-capillary network* which allowed so much fresh air to be absorbed by the blood in such a short time. In the second volume of these essays, published in 1735 he reported measurements made by direct observation on the rate of blood flow in the lung capillaries of frogs, from which he concluded that the blood must pass through the lung very much more rapidly than through other parts of the body.

Up to that time the composition of air was unknown and there-fore it could not be appreciated that only part of the air is essential

*The interconnecting network of capillaries and air sacs in the lungs.

for breathing. Knowledge of this had to wait until developments in chemical methods enabled gases to be analysed. The Scottish chemist Joseph Black, in 1757, showed that when heated carbonates lose weight with the liberation of a gas called by him 'fixed air' later to be known as carbon dioxide. Eight years after this Henry Cavendish, the eccentric philosopher, by the action of acid on certain metals, isolated another gas, called by him 'inflammable air', later to be known as hydrogen. Analysis of atmospheric air itself was carried out by Joseph Priestley, a Presbyterian minister in Leeds and a self-taught chemist, whose interest in gases was aroused by the fumes emanating from a near-by brewery. On 1 August 1774 he isolated a gas which he called 'dephlogisticated air' by heating mercuric red oxide in a closed container. He found that a candle burnt in this gas, later to be known as oxygen, with a remarkably vigorous flame and that a piece of red-hot wood glowed brightly and burnt rapidly. In March 1775 he showed that mice lived longer in a container filled with this new gas than in an equal volume of atmospheric air. Shortly afterwards he identified a second gas from the atmosphere, which, later known as nitrogen, he called 'phlogisticated air'. His choice of name for these two constituents of air arose from the theory current at that time that a hypothetical substance called 'phlogiston' was liberated from all combustible materials during combustion. Priestley therefore believed that atmospheric air, during respiration, lost its phlogiston and it was this dephlogisticated air that was essential for the maintenance of life.

His scientific work came to an end in 1791 when, living in Birmingham, his home was burned down by an angry mob protesting against his support of the French Revolution which he had demonstrated by

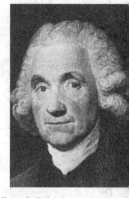

Joseph Priestley
(1733–1804)

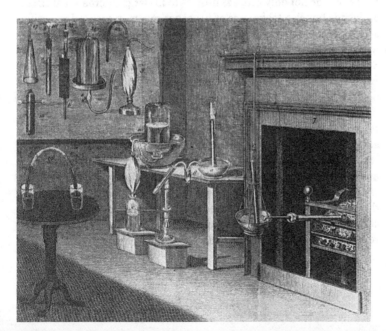

Chemical apparatus
used by Joseph Priestley
for his experiments
on fixed air

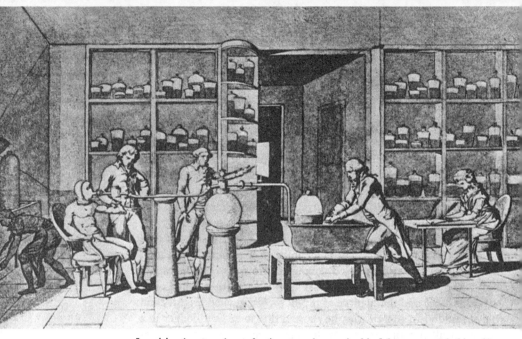

Lavoisier (1743–94) conducting experiments in his laboratory with his wife taking notes seated at the table

joining with friends in celebrating the second anniversary of Bastille Day. Two years later he left England to join his sons in Pennsylvania where he became a Unitarian minister.

Antoine Laurent Lavoisier, the Parisian financier, politician and scientist, became interested in the problems of respiration after he had studied a translation of the second edition of Priestley's book on this subject and had met him on a visit to Paris in 1774, the year he isolated dephlogisticated air. Lavoisier was greatly assisted in this work by a devoted wife whom he had married when she was only fourteen: she not only acted as hostess to his large international circle of friends but also took notes of his experiments, translated scientific articles and engraved illustrations for his publications. His research work in chemistry began when he was elected to the Académie des Sciences in 1768 at the age of twenty-five, and continued at the Arsenal, the state-controlled centre for the manufacture of gunpowder where he built a laboratory in 1775. In 1772 he showed that sulphur and phosphorus on being burnt gain weight due, he said, to the addition of prodigious quantities of air. He referred to this again at the Easter meeting of the Académie three years later when he said, 'the principle combining with metals during their calcination and augmenting their weight is nothing else than the pure portion of air which surrounds us and which we breathe'. He realised that this was the same as Priestley's dephlogisticated air but being aware of the absurdity of the phlogiston theory called it instead the eminently respirable air and later oxygen. Further, he showed that when a metal in combination with oxygen is reduced to its original form, in the presence of charcoal, the carbon joins with the oxygen to form Black's 'fixed air' or what Priestley called carbon dioxide. It was his identification of oxygen in the inspired air and carbon dioxide in the expired air, which led to his belief that respiration was a slow form of combustion. On 3 May 1777 he read an essay to the Académie in which he pointed out that inspired air is composed of the eminently respirable portion and another passive component later to be known as nitrogen. At first he thought that this process of combustion took place in the lungs themselves with carbon, brought there by the blood, reacting with the oxygen from the air to form carbon dioxide; and that the heat resulting from this reaction was distributed by the blood to maintain the body temperature. Later however, he began to have doubts whether the process was confined to the lungs and in 1790 suggested that possibly it also took place in other parts of the body. He was not able to develop this idea further but his contributions were of the greatest importance and his numerous painstaking experiments which formed the basis of modern chemistry were described in his classic *Elementary Treatise on Chemistry* published in 1789. Lavoisier was unfortunately a victim of the French Revolution, and was guillotined on 8 May 1794 at the age of fifty. Lagrange, the mathematician, hearing of his death exclaimed, 'it took only one moment to sever that head, and perhaps a century will not be enough to produce another like it'.

It was nearly half a century after his death before the German, Gustav Magnus, by determining and comparing the oxygen and carbon dioxide content of the veins and arteries, correctly recognised that combustion takes place in all the tissues of the body. The complete understanding of the mechanism by which gases are transported in the body has only been achieved during the past hundred years. Germans, such as Otto Funke, Lothar Meyer, Carl Ludwig and F. Hoppe-Seyler, were the first to show, about the middle of the last century, that oxygen is carried in the blood by the protein haemoglobin contained in the red blood cells. The effect of carbon dioxide pressure on the binding of oxygen by haemoglobin was demonstrated early in this century in Copenhagen by Christian Bohr, August Krogh and K. A. Hasselbalch. Bohr, unfortunately, was misled into thinking that there must be an active secretion of oxygen by the lungs into the blood. His student, August Krogh, aided by his wife Marie, had shown by 1910 that the oxygen pressure is always higher in the air sacs of the lungs than in arterial blood and that diffusion alone is enough to explain pulmonary gas exchange.

The further study of the chemistry of the blood in relation to the respiratory gases was next developed by the British-American school of respiratory physiologists which included John Scott Haldane (1860–1936) Joseph Barcroft (1872–1947) and Lawrence J. Henderson (1878–1942).

It was Haldane's interest in the problems of coal miners and the gases to which they are exposed which led to his interest in respiration. Joseph Barcroft, the Cambridge physiologist, increased our knowledge of the principles underlying oxygen absorption. He discovered different kinds of haemoglobin and demonstrated the effects of high and low altitudes upon the blood gases. It was Henderson and his associates at Harvard, together with Donald Van Slyke and his colleagues at the Rockefeller Institute in New York, in the years immediately after the First World War, who finally worked out the exact relationship and interreaction between the various electrolytes and gases found in the blood and the tissues.

Our present knowledge of the transport and exchange of gases in the body may be summarised as follows. The normal person respires about a thousand millilitres of air a minute during which time approximately two hundred and fifty millilitres of oxygen pass into the blood and two hundred and fifty millilitres of carbon dioxide are liberated into the lungs. A similar exchange takes place in reverse in the tissues. The movement of gases between the blood and the alveolar air, and between the blood and the tissues, is basically due to diffusion from points of higher pressure to points of lower pressure. The pressure exerted by a gas in a mixture of gases is called its partial pressure. The partial pressure of oxygen in the alveoli is a hundred millimetres of mercury whereas in the blood arriving in the lung capillaries it is only forty millimetres of mercury and, because of this, oxygen diffuses from the alveoli to the blood through the alveolar-capillary membrane. The partial pressure of carbon dioxide in the venous blood reaching the lungs is forty-six millimetres of mercury compared with forty millimetres of mercury in alveolar air so that the carbon dioxide diffuses from the blood into the alveoli. Similar pressure relationships control gaseous diffusion in and out of the tissues.

The liquid part of blood, the plasma, is a very poor carrier of oxygen, with only a very small fraction dissolved in it, whereas the protein haemoglobin in the red cells rapidly combines with most of the oxygen so that in the lungs it becomes 90 per cent saturated, forming the compound oxyhaemoglobin. The carbon dioxide formed by tissue metabolism diffuses into the blood plasma and from there passes into the red cells where about four-fifths of it reacts with water under the influence of the enzyme carbonic anhydrase to form carbonic acid. The carbonic acid immediately splits into hydrogen and bicarbonate ions, the latter being transported to the lungs in combination with potassium (and to a lesser extent with sodium) in the cells. The remaining fifth combines with reduced haemoglobin.

The transport of these gases to and from the tissues therefore depends on the proper functioning of the lungs, heart and blood. Patients with lung disease, heart failure or anaemia, because of difficulty in getting oxygen to their tissues, suffer from shortness of breath, or dyspnoea (from the Greek *dus*—bad, and *pneo*—breathe.) Cyanosis, the distinctive bluish colour of the skin, is caused by an excess amount of non-oxygenated haemoglobin in the capillaries and is therefore seen in respiratory disease and cardiac failure but not in anaemia where the haemoglobin is in short supply.

5

The structure and function of the heart

THE anatomy and physiology of the heart will be briefly reviewed as a basis for the proper understanding of developments in knowledge of its disorders and their treatment since the time of Harvey.

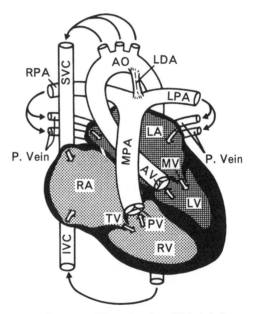

The normal heart. AO, aorta; AV aortic valve; IVC, inferior vena cava; LA, left atrium; LPA, left pulmonary artery; LV, left ventricle; MPA, main pulmonary artery; MV, mitral valve; LDA, ligamentum ductus arteriosus; PV, pulmonary valve; P vein, pulmonary vein; RA, right atrium; RPA, right pulmonary artery; RV, right ventricle; SVC, superior vena cava; TV, tricuspid valve

The heart is a hollow muscular organ which, as may be seen from the radiograph of the chest lies behind the sternum or breast-bone between the two lungs, so that it is far more in the centre of the

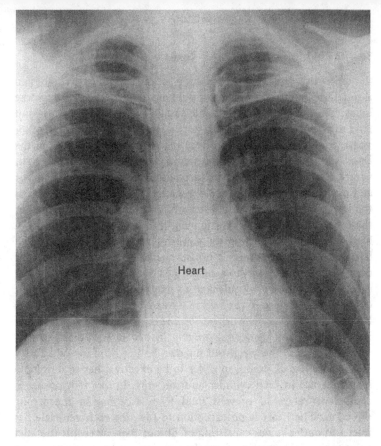

Heart

Chest radiograph. The heart, bones and bloodvessels cast white shadows in contrast to the lungs, extending from the root of the neck to the diaphragm, which appear black

chest than most people imagine. It is divided by a wall or septum into a right and left half, each half being divided again into an upper and lower part. The upper chambers, now known as the atria were, until recent years, called auricles,* a term now reserved for the smaller, ear-like appendages which project forwards from each atrium. The walls of the atria are composed of a thin layer of muscle, unlike the walls of the lower chambers or ventricles, which are very much thicker, particularly of the left ventricle. Blood from the upper and lower parts of the body drains into the right atrium through two great veins, the superior and inferior vena cava. From the right atrium it flows into the right ventricle where it is pumped through the pulmonary artery into the lungs. Blood from the lungs passes through the pulmonary veins to the left atrium and thence into the left ventricle, which pumps it into the great artery, or aorta, whose branches divide and subdivide throughout the body. There are,

*In this book the terms atria and auricles will be employed interchangeably according to the historical context.

therefore, two separate circulations, a greater or systemic circulation through the body, and a lesser or pulmonary circulation through the lungs. The purpose of the systemic circulation is to carry oxygen and food to all parts of the body and to remove carbon dioxide and other waste products of metabolism from the tissues. The purpose of the lesser circulation is to carry deoxygenated blood from the right ventricle to the lungs where its carbon dioxide is liberated to the air and oxygen absorbed, so that oxygenated blood may be supplied to the left side of the heart for distribution to the body. The blood in these two circulations is kept moving by the heart which acts as a highly efficient and extremely powerful two-cylinder pump. The left ventricle at rest exerts a pressure sufficient to lift a weight of over 2 oz (approx. 56 g) to a height of 5 ft (1·5 m) or more so that each hour it does work equivalent to that required to raise a weight of approximately 500 lb (227 kg) to the same height. From this it has been calculated that the work performed in twenty-four hours by the left ventricle in a man lying quietly in bed is equivalent to that required to raise the weight of his own body to the top of a forty-storey building. A pump, in order to be effective, has to develop a high pressure in each cylinder and can only do this if it possesses competent valves to prevent fluid from escaping in the wrong direction. The heart is no exception to this, for each ventricle has inlet and outlet valves consisting of fibrous flaps or cusps; the inlet valve to the right ventricle from the right atrium has three cusps and is thus called the tricuspid valve whereas the one at the opening into the left ventricle has only two cusps and from its shape like that of a bishop's mitre is called the mitral valve. Thin strong cords, known as chordae tendinae, like the ropes of a parachute, connect the under surface of the cusps of these inlet valves to the walls of the ventricles where they are tethered to short muscular pillars known as the papillary muscles. The purpose of these cords is not to close the valves but to prevent them from billowing upwards into the atria when the ventricles contract. The valves are closed by the rise in pressure which occurs within the cavity of each ventricle when it starts to undergo contraction. As the pressure rises still higher, the two outlet valves, the pulmonary valve and the aortic valve, which consist of three strong fibrous cusps (but without chordae tendinae) situated at the mouths of the pulmonary artery and aorta respectively, are forced open and remain open until relaxation of the ventricles causes the pressure within these chambers to fall below that in the two main arteries, when the valves close. The pressure in the ventricles then continues to fall until it is below that in the atria when the valves between the chambers open and allow blood once again to fill the ventricles. This cardiac cycle repeated about seventy times a minute is associated with two audible sounds phonetically represented by 'lubb-dup'. The first sound, 'lubb', is caused by closure of the mitral and tricuspid valves, the second one, 'dup', by the closure of the aortic and pulmonary valves. The interval, therefore, between the first and second sounds is the time during which the ventricles are in a state of contraction or systole and the interval between the second and the first sounds, the time when, in their relaxed state, or diastole, they fill with blood from the atria. Additional sounds called murmurs are heard when disease interferes with the flow of blood. The amount of blood ejected during each ventricular systole is approximately 60 ml per ventricle so that the total cardiac output is approximately 3·5–5 litres a minute at rest; a healthy man can increase this to over 20 litres a minute during very strenuous exercise. The muscle of the ventricles, in order to accomplish this, has to be extremely powerful and well nourished with blood which is supplied by two coronary arteries rising from the mouth of the aorta. These are long slender vessels which divide and subdivide through-out the substance of the muscle; their branches are linked by a net-work of vessels which in health are closed and only open when one of the main channels becomes blocked by disease, to form an alter-native collateral circulation.

The heart's action is controlled by nerves connected to the brain and by chemical substances in the circulation. Both mechanisms are constantly in operation so as to ensure the most appropriate response of the organ on all occasions. The nervous control is brought about by the action of the parasympathetic and sympathetic components of the autonomic nervous system.* Parasympathetic nerve impulses in the vagus nerve slow the heart whilst those in sympathetic nerve fibres increase its rate so that these two different types of nerve act as a brake and an accelerator respectively. Special nerve endings, responsive to changes in pressure, are found in the great veins and right atrium so that when the circulation becomes inadequate for the body's needs, such as in health during violent exercise or in disease when the heart fails, the increased pressure of the blood which accumulates on the venous side acts on these nerve endings with the setting up of impulses which affect the cardiac control centres in the brain. These in turn inhibit the action of the vagus whilst increasing the activity of the sympathetic nerve, thus causing a com-pensatory increase in heart rate and output. Similar nerve endings are found in the walls of the aorta and the internal carotid artery, which, when stimulated by a rise in arterial pressure, have an

*Autonomic nervous system: that part of the nervous system which is largely independent of the central nervous system and controls the action of ductless glands, blood vessels, and all organs containing involuntary muscle.

opposite effect on the cardiac control centres with an appropriate adjustment of the autonomic nervous system and diminution of the cardiac rate and output. Other factors which influence the heart's action include fever, thyroxin from the thyroid gland, adrenalin from the adrenal gland and lack of oxygen, all of which increase the heart's action. Emotions also often cause the heart to beat faster although sudden shock may slow it, or even temporarily stop it, with consequent fainting.

Arteries have a similar innervation to the heart with sympathetic and parasympathetic fibres of the autonomic nervous system under the control of vasomotor centres* adjacent to the cardiac centres in

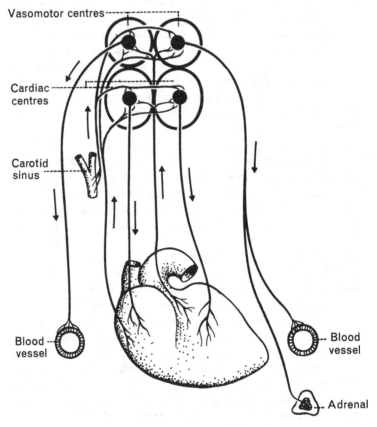

Sympathetic and parasympathetic nerves linking the autonomic centres in the brain with the heart and bloodvessels

*The vasomotor centres regulate the contraction of vessels (vasoconstriction) and their expansion (vasodilatation).

the brain. This allows appropriate adjustments in the calibre of the vessels to be made, at the same time as alterations in the speed and force of the heart's action occur in response to the body's requirements. Physical exertion for example requires an increase in cardiac output, with a rise in arterial blood pressure in order to provide an increased circulation of blood to the muscles. This is achieved by the brain stimulating the adrenal glands to liberate adrenalin into the circulation whilst at the same time increasing the activity of the sympathetic nervous system. The combination of these two actions results in an increased heart rate and constriction of the arteries to most organs of the body, with an associated rise in arterial blood pressure. The blood vessels in the muscles however instead of constricting, undergo dilatation as a direct result of the effect on them of accumulated metabolites resulting from their increased activity. The effect of these vessels being dilated at the same time as the blood pressure in general is raised, is to increase the blood flow through the muscles, thus providing them with sufficient oxygen for their needs and removing the waste products of their metabolism. The elevation of the blood pressure is kept within safe limits by the effect it exerts on the nerve endings in the aorta and carotid arteries connected to the vasomotor centres in the brain which, when the pressure rises too high, reduces it by adjusting the action of the autonomic nervous system on the heart and blood vessels.

Most of our knowledge of the various mechanisms by which control is exerted over the action of the heart and the circulation of the blood has been acquired within about the last two hundred years. The French physician, Jean-Baptiste de Sénac, in his book on the structure, function and diseases of the heart in 1749, gave a far more detailed account of the anatomy and physiology of the organ than had appeared in any previous work. In the second edition, published in 1777, he drew attention to the way in which arteries undergo alternate contractions and dilatations similar to the movements of the heart. The German, Weber, in 1831, first showed that the movements of the arteries and the heart are controlled by the same type of special nerves and in 1840 the German physiologist, Stelling, first referred to these nerves acting on the arteries as 'vasomotor nerves', a term which came into general use after the publication of important papers on the subject by Claude Bernard, Brown-Séquard and Augustus Waller, ten years later.

Claude Bernard was the greatest of the French physiologists. His discovery of the function of the vasomotor nerves was only one of his many contributions and arose from work he did on the role of the sympathetic nerves in regulating the metabolism and in controlling the temperature of the body. Included in his famous experiments was his observation, published in 1852, that division of the sympathetic nerves in the neck of a rabbit causes elevation of the temperature and an increase in the circulation of the affected side of the face and ear. He and his friend, Charles Brown-Séquard, received their training in Paris from François Magendie who was the chief clinician at the Hôtel-Dieu there and professor at the Collège de France where he conducted experiments in physiology and pharmacology. He showed much interest in his pupils' work on the nervous control of the cardiovascular system and used to discuss the progress of their experiments with them at weekly meetings of the Societé de Biologie in Paris. Brown-Séquard's experiments, also published in 1852, showed that, whilst cutting the sympathetic nerve evoked vasodilatation, stimulation of peripheral sympathetic nerve endings induced vasoconstriction, a phenomenon also described by the English physiologist, Augustus Waller, one year later. About the same time Claude Bernard in France and Schiff in Germany, on the basis of experiments that involved cutting the brain stem and spinal cord of animals at different levels, demonstrated the presence of the special vasomotor control centres in the brain. Little was known,

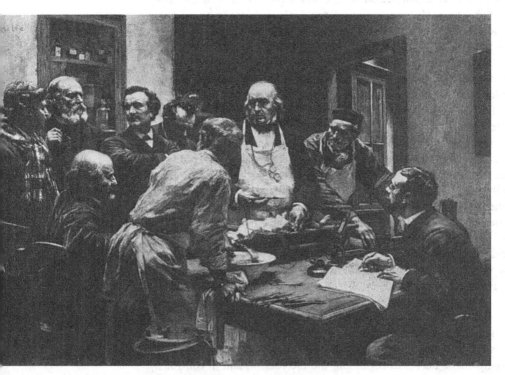

Claude Bernard demonstrating an experiment.

however, as to what influenced their action until Yandell Henderson, in America, showed in 1907 that one important factor was variations in the carbon dioxide pressure in the circulation.

Physiology is indebted to W. H. Gaskell and J. N. Langley, both of whom worked at Cambridge, for the proper understanding of the autonomic nervous system and the interrelationship between the

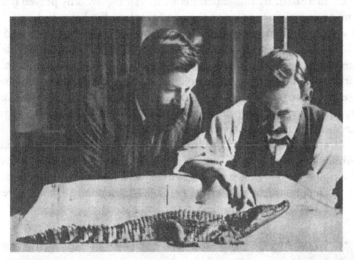

W. H. Gaskell (1847–1914) with his 'lab-boy' Thomas Metcalfe on his left. In the foreground is one of the crocodiles on which Gaskell worked out the autonomic nerve supply to the heart

parasympathetic and sympathetic systems acting on the various parts of the body, including the heart and blood vessels. Gaskell summarised the results of his work in his book *The Involuntary Nervous System* published in 1920; and Langley summarised his in *The Autonomic Nervous System* published in 1921. Research into the problem of how the autonomic nerve fibres act on tissue cells was begun by T. R. Elliott, a student in the Department of Physiology at Cambridge, whose recognition of the similarity between the action of adrenalin from the adrenal glands and of the sympathetic nerves led him, in 1904, to propose that adrenalin or a related substance might be released at the sympathetic nerve endings. This work was continued by Henry Dale (later Sir Henry Dale), an outstanding pupil of Gaskell and Langley, when he was at Cambridge, and by Otto Loewi, Professor of Pharmacology at Graz. Loewi, in 1921, removed the hearts from two frogs, the first with the nerves intact and the second without. Life in the hearts was maintained by perfusing them with a special electrolytic fluid known as Ringer's solution. The parasympathetic fibres of the vagus nerve attached to

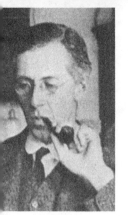

Sir Henry Dale
(1875–1968)

the first heart were stimulated for a few minutes. Then the Ringer solution in that heart was transferred to the second one with the effect that its action slowed and its beats diminished just as if its vagus had been stimulated. Similarly, when the sympathetic nerve fibres of the first heart were stimulated and the surrounding Ringer's solution transferred to the second heart the latter's speed and activity were increased. By this experiment Loewi unequivocally proved that the autonomic nerves exert their influence on the heart and vessels by the liberation of specific chemical substances. Dale had already shown, in 1914, that the substance released at the parasympathetic nerve endings is acetyl choline, and subsequent work by him and others has shown that it is also liberated by sympathetic vasodilator nerve fibres whilst an adrenalin-like substance is produced at sympathetic vasoconstrictor nerve endings. For his contribution to medical science Dale was awarded the Nobel Prize in 1936.

No account of the physiology of the heart would be complete without reference to William Bayliss (1860–1924) and Ernest Starling (1856–1927) who worked together on important animal experiments when at University College, London. Shortly after

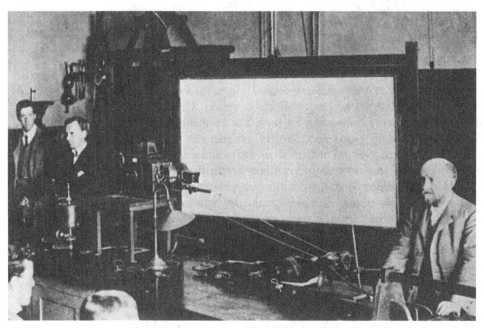

One of the photographs presented in court in the Brown Dog Case. This shows William Bayliss performing an experiment and to his right beyond the screen is Ernest Starling and beside him H. Dale (later Sir Henry Dale)

Bayliss had become head of the Physiology Department there in 1903 the entire country became engrossed in following the course of a libel and slander action taken by him against the Hon. Stephen Coleridge, secretary of an anti-vivisection society, who had made accusations against Bayliss and Starling of cruelty in their treatment of dogs during experiments. The verdict in favour of Bayliss on 18 November 1903, was received in court with loud and prolonged applause and the sum of £2,000 awarded to him he gave to his department which, having invested it wisely, still profits from the interest. Starling's investigation of cardiac function with a special isolated heart/lung preparation of a mammalian heart led to important advances in our knowledge of cardiac control and his 'law of the heart' is familiar to all students of physiology.

6

Simultaneous attack on the joints and the heart

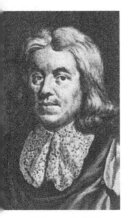

*Thomas Sydenham
(1624–89)*

ACUTE rheumatic fever, a disease in which transitory pains in the joints are often followed by severe damage to the heart, was at one time a common childhood disorder. It arises as a complication of streptococcal infection in the throat. Since the introduction of penicillin twenty-five years ago and its use in the treatment of streptococcal infections, the incidence of rheumatic fever has fallen dramatically so that now a medical student might complete his training without seeing more than the occasional child affected by it. There is, however, still a large number of adults suffering from the long-term effects of the disease on the heart; fortunately many of these patients can now be helped by cardiac surgery.

Rheumatism, originally a generic term for all types of pain affecting the musculo-skeletal system, has regrettably continued to be used in this sense up to the present time, often as a cloak for ignorance, despite Thomas Sydenham's attempt in his *Medical Observations*, published in 1676, to reserve it specifically for the characteristic involvement of the joints in the disease now known as acute rheumatic fever. In a chapter entitled 'Rheumatism' he said:

The sad list of symptoms begins with chills and shivers ... one or two days after this the patient is attacked by severe pains in the joints, sometimes in one and sometimes in another, sometimes in his wrists, sometimes in his shoulder, sometimes in the knee ... this pain changes its place from time to time, takes the joints in turn and affects the ones that it attacks last with redness and swelling.

This clear description of rheumatic fever as it affects the joints, although written in the seventeenth century, could not be bettered today. His ability to write lucid descriptions of several important diseases was because, like Hippocrates whom he greatly admired, he was a skilled observer. His rejoinder to Sir Hans Sloane, who in his youth was given a testimonial describing him as a good botanist and skilful anatomist, was, 'anatomy, botany, nonsense! No, young man, go to the bedside; there alone can you learn disease!'

Thomas Sydenham (1624–89) born at Wynford Eagle in Dorset of a rich Puritan family, had his studies at Oxford interrupted when, in the Civil War, he enlisted in Cromwell's army and served for four years as captain of a troop of horse. His return to Oxford in 1647 was followed only six months later by the Earl of Pembroke, Chancellor of the University, taking the somewhat unprecedented and highly irregular step of having him created a Bachelor of Medicine. However, his studies continued at Montpellier under Charles Barbeyrac, a medical teacher of great repute.

Sydenham started practice in London in 1661, at a time when medicine was bogged down by nebulous theories, hypotheses and speculations. He freed himself entirely from these and by a careful study of the pattern of disease laid the foundations of modern clinical medicine. His methods of treatment were logical and practical in an age, according to one writer, John Brown, when they were 'over-run and stultified by vile and silly nostrums'. Like Hippocrates, who taught that nature often terminates disease spontaneously without the help of medicine, Sydenham said that in many cases 'I have consulted my patients' safety and my own reputation most effectually by doing nothing at all'.

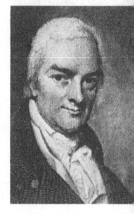

John Haygarth
(1740–1827)

It was not until after his death that his clinical methods and writings received their deserved acclaim. In 1810, one hundred and twenty-one years after his death, the Royal College of Physicians recognised that his achievements marked an epoch in the history of medicine and a tablet to his memory was erected in St James's Church, Piccadilly, where he is buried.

Another English physician who made an important contribution to our knowledge of rheumatic fever was John Haygarth (1740–1827) who in 1805 when a consulting physician at the Infirmary in Chester published an account *Of the Acute Rheumatism or Rheumatick Fever*. In this review of 10,549 patients in his practice he said:

The term rheumatism both in common and medical language includes a great variety of disorders which ought to be distinguished from each other by different names. After separating it from the nodosity of the joints, tic douloureux, sciatica, lumbago, and other diseases which nosologists have placed under this denomination, there still remain 470 cases of rheumatism. This disease is generally classed with fevers and yet only 170 had any fever. These last are the cases which come under the title of acute rheumatism and exclusively form the subject of the following pages.

In his subsequent account he described the fever and characteristic involvement of the joints in a similar manner to Sydenham, at the same time emphasising that in his opinion exposure to cold and moisture is a principal cause of the disease.

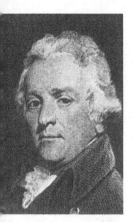

David Pitcairn
(1749–1809)

The joint changes and fever of acute rheumatic fever were therefore well known by the end of the eighteenth century. Also about that time others drew attention to the cardiac complications of the disease. Dr David Pitcairn, a physician at St Bartholomew's Hospital, London, although he did not write on the subject, was teaching his students about this complication by 1788. At a meeting of the Fleece Medical Society, which took its name from The Fleece Inn, Rodborough, Gloucestershire, where it met, Edward Jenner the country general practitioner best known for his introduction of vaccination, drew the attention of the Society, in 1789, to a disease of the heart following acute rheumatism. But it was not until William Charles Wells discussed the subject in lectures in London that it became widely recognised.

Wells started life in Charleston, South Carolina, his father, a bookseller and bookbinder, having emigrated there from Scotland in 1753. Because of his father's affection for his native land young Wells was sent back to Scotland to attend the grammar school in Dumfries, followed by a year at the University of Edinburgh. In 1771 he returned to Charleston to serve an apprenticeship with Dr Alexander Garden, whose name has been perpetuated by the celebrated botanist Linnaeus who named what he considered to be one of the most beautiful flowering shrubs, the gardenia, in honour of this physician.

At the outbreak of the War of Independence, Wells and his father left America and in 1776 he continued his medical studies first in Edinburgh and later at St Bartholomew's Hospital in London. Soon after qualification he had to give up medicine for a time in order to go back to South Carolina to settle his father's business which had been mismanaged by an elder brother. For a time he then earned his living as a bookseller, supplemented by acting in a local theatre in Florida until forced to spend three months in prison in Charleston because of his brother's debts.

He arrived once again in London in May 1784, where he started a medical practice; became Physician to the Finsbury Dispensary in 1789 and a physician at St Thomas's Hospital in 1800. Unfortunately during that year he had his first attack of apoplexy but, by strict dieting, managed to keep himself in fair health for several years until in 1813, he began to show signs of heart failure from which he died on 18 September 1817. In spite of his poor health he wrote many scientific papers including an important one on the cardiac complications of rheumatic fever published in 1810. In this paper entitled 'On Rheumatism of the Heart', he acknowledged the teaching of Dr David Pitcairn and described fourteen cases, including nine of his own patients and five of his colleagues.

Rheumatic fever, when it affects the heart, causes damage to the muscle and the valves, also in severe cases involves the outer covering or pericardium. The changes in the muscle lead to an increase in the force and speed of the heart's action which, when particularly severe, causes distressing palpitations. And the pericarditis, when present, is accompanied by severe chest pain. It was the occurrence of one or both of these symptoms in patients who a short time previously had suffered from rheumatic fever affecting the joints, that drew Wells's attention to the heart complications in this disease.

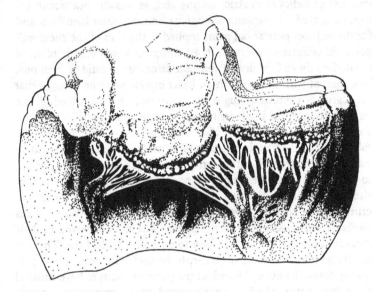

Rheumatic vegetations consisting of a bead-like row of warty nodules on the cusps of the mitral valve

The important changes in the valves which are obvious on listening to the heart were not recognised by him as the stethoscope had not yet been invented. It is interesting too that although from his descriptions his cases were obviously extremely severe and many of them quickly passed into irreversible heart failure he did not mention in his reports of six cases examined after death any damage to the valves or, in particular, the presence of the characteristic vegetations commonly found on the valves in this disease.

It is now known that changes in the joints may range from being so mild as to be overlooked, to such severity as to cause temporary crippling, but they rarely leave residual damage, unlike the heart changes which, when they occur, are often permanent. For this reason it has been said that it is a disease 'which licks the joints, but bites the heart'.

Treatment of this disease in the early nineteenth century was most unsatisfactory. Admittedly Wells gave his patients bed-rest and prescribed laudanum, a preparation of opium popularised by Sydenham, which must have been useful in the treatment of heart failure and have relieved the pain arising from the joints and the inflamed pericardium; also, he used digitalis, a most valuable drug in the management of heart failure even though its indications and dosage had not been properly established in his time. Most of his other measures must only have added considerably to the patients' distress; he believed in strict dieting and, as was the practice in his day, subjected his patients to copious and repeated bleedings and for the relief of pericardial pain, applied to the skin of the chest wall powerful counter-irritants, such as cantharides, sufficiently often to break the skin and produce a constant discharge of fluid or even pus. Not content with this, in cases of heart involvement he thought that the cardiac condition might be improved by transferring the inflammation to the joints by the application of cantharides to them. In discussing this method of treatment in one case he said, 'I followed this practice in the case of Miss A.L., but she suffered so much distress from the stimulating substances, which were applied to her joints, that her mother soon removed them and, as her situation had from the first appeared to be hopeless, I thought it cruel to urge their renewal'. He was well aware that many of his methods were distressing to the patient but as he believed in their efficacy considered it was his duty to persevere with them. Thus, in his discussion of two of his patients he said, 'In both of the preceding cases, the general health of the patients seems to have suffered from the means which were employed to overcome the internal inflammation; but, I shall not hence be deterred, from using the same means in an equal degree, in any similar case that may hereafter occur to me'.

Satisfactory treatment of the pain and inflammation in the joints was not obtained until the discovery of salicylates. Cinchona bark, which contains quinine, was imported from Peru by Sydenham in the seventeenth century for the treatment of ague or malaria, a very common disease in this country at that time. This drug was expensive and, as it was considered that wherever a disease was prevalent nature would always provide a remedy and as willow trees and malaria both occurred in marshy places, willow bark which contains salacin came to be used as a cheap substitute for imported cinchona in all types of fever by the next century. When in the latter half of the nineteenth century salicylates were developed from salacin and found to be effective not only in reducing fever but also in counteracting pain sodium salicylate was introduced for the treatment of rheumatic fever. Salicylates are so effective in controlling the joint symptoms in acute rheumatic fever that they bring relief within forty-eight hours. At one time it was thought that they also helped to protect the heart but this now seems unlikely; in fact, it has been shown that the progress of children who develop cardiac failure during an acute attack is made worse by their administration. Since 1948 cortisone and allied substances have been used in the treatment of rheumatic fever. There is no doubt that they provide dramatic relief of the pain in the joints and it is possible, but not certain, that they may prevent the development of late cardiac complications but as, however, they have certain important side effects many authorities advocate that their use should be reserved for cases already in established heart failure or suffering from the severe pain of peri-carditis.

Rheumatic fever has always been found to be most prevalent in children living in a cold damp climate and subjected to overcrowding and poverty. For a long time it was thought that the disease must be caused by an infection resulting from direct invasion of the joints and heart with bacteria, but repeated attempts to isolate infective organisms from these structures were unsuccessful. It was then observed by Bernard Schlesinger in England in 1930, and by Alvin F. Coburn in America in 1931, that epidemics of sore throats due to infection with the Lancefield group A type of haemolytic streptococcus were always followed by an increase in the number of cases of rheumatic fever in the community; also that whether the disease occurred sporadically or during an epidemic it invariably appeared two to three weeks after the sore throat. It only arises, however, in a minority of people so that in an epidemic it is seen in about 3 per cent of those at risk. The characteristic changes in the joints and heart are now considered to be some type of allergic reaction to the throat organisms and only occur in people with a herditary predisposition. Fortunately penicillin readily kills streptococci and since its introduction in the early part of the Second World War throat infections due to this organism have been easily cured and their spread prevented. This has led to a dramatic decrease in the number of cases of rheumatic fever. Also, the recurrence of the disease with its risk of further cardiac damage may be prevented by giving a child, after the first attack, a small number of penicillin tablets every day until adult life is reached so that any further throat infections may be avoided. This prophylactic measure is extremely valuable but one which at times has proved to be disappointing in practice as it is difficult to get fit children to remember to take their tablets regularly. The expectation of life for patients affected by the disease has also been much improved by the spectacular advances in surgery during the last twenty years which have made possible the replacement or repair of damaged valves.

The annual death rate from rheumatic fever in England and Wales dropped from 67 per million in 1901 to 23 per million in 1939 on account of improvements in living conditions alone and, with the introduction of penicillin, it was by 1965 only 2 per million. An interesting survey conducted on behalf of the Scottish Health Services Council and published in 1967 shows that routine inspection of school-children in that country revealed 361 cases of acquired heart disease (in that context rheumatic fever) per 100,000 in 1949 but only 95 per 100,000 in 1964, also that the death rate from rheumatic cardiac damage fell from 1 per 100,000 of the population in 1954 to only 0·1 per 100,000 in 1963.

7

The foxglove as a therapeutic weapon

AN outstanding advance in the treatment of heart disease occurred in the eighteenth century when the importance of a drug called digitalis was recognised by William Withering. Withering was born in Wellington, Shropshire, in 1741; his grandfather, father and uncle were all physicians, so from an early age he was in close contact with the profession he himself was ultimately to follow. After a private education, he studied medicine at the University of Edinburgh before entering general practice in Stafford in 1767. There, in addition to his routine medical duties, he found time to make a detailed study of the plants in the neighbourhood and his systematically compiled notes of this formed the basis of his first book, *A Botanical arrangement of all the Vegetables naturally growing in Great Britain*, published in 1776. The previous year he had left Stafford, where he was earning on an average only £100 per annum and moved to Birmingham where, after the first year, his income had increased to over £1,000 a year. His practice there was so successful, and his patients scattered over such a wide area, that a light was installed in his carriage to enable him to continue his studies while travelling. His scientific interests were not confined to botany and medicine: he also became an expert chemist with a special interest in minerals. It was his discovery of barium carbonate which led Werner, the German geologist, to name the substance Witherite. He was a member of the select Lunar Society, a scientific body which in his time included Joseph Priestley and James Watt.

In 1775 Withering's opinion was sought as to the value of a recipe kept secret for a long time by an old woman in Shropshire who had used it as a cure for dropsy, often when doctors had failed. He was told that it caused violent purging and vomiting and that it was considered that this was the reason for its effectiveness. From Withering's examination of the twenty or more herbs in the remedy he concluded that only the foxglove could be the active ingredient: exactly how he knew this is not made clear, although of course as a

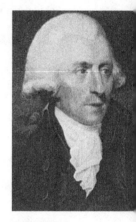

William Withering (1741–99)

botanist he was well acquainted with the foxglove, or digitalis, so named by Fuchsius in 1542 in allusion to the German *Fingerhüt*—finger stall—from the resemblance of the blossom to the fingers of a glove.

Withering decided to try the effect of this substance on the sick poor who attended his house in Birmingham. He said:

My worthy predecessor in this place, the very humane and ingenious Dr Small, had made it a practise to give his advice to the poor during one hour in a day. This practise, which I continued until we had a hospital open for the reception of the sick poor, gave me an opportunity of putting my ideas into execution in a variety of cases; for the number of poor who thus applied for advice, amounted to between two and three thousand annually.

He admits that when he first used the drug, because of the pressure of work he did not keep any notes, but formed the definite impression that it was helpful in relieving dropsy. Shrewdly he realised that the beneficial effect was not so much due to vomiting and purging as to a diuretic* effect on the kidneys. At first he refrained from using it on his more influential patients, until he heard from a colleague, Dr Ash, that the Principal of Brasenose College, Oxford, a sufferer from heart failure, had derived much benefit from administration of the plant's root. This encouraged him to use it more widely and to study in greater detail the best type of preparation and optimum dosage. Aware that it was essential to standardise the drug in order to avoid unpredictable effects, he thought that instead of using the root it would be better to use the leaves, but as their potency varied at different seasons he decided to use them only when the plant was in flower. He dried the leaves in the sun, or by placing them in a pan over a fire, and the resultant green powder was administered either alone or in the form of pills by the addition of soap. At other times, when a liquid was preferred, he made an infusion by steeping the dried leaves in boiling water.

An opportunity to further his experience in the use of the drug occurred in 1779 when he had a large number of cases of heart failure in his practice. They must have been the result of rheumatic fever, as he says that they followed an epidemic of scarlet fever and sore throat in the area. He achieved such spectacular success with the drug that a friend, Dr Stokes, reported his results to the Medical Society at Edinburgh and in consequence the drug became widely used in the Infirmary there and appeared in the *Edinburgh Pharmacopoeia* in 1783. Withering however became dismayed at the excessive dosage employed both in Edinburgh and London for he was certain that if this practice continued the drug would soon fall into

*Diuretic, from the Greek *diouretikos*—(adj.) increasing the secretion of urine; (n) a substance that promotes the secretion of urine.

disrepute because of its unpleasant side effects. In an effort to avoid this he decided to write a book, setting out his experiences with the drug, for as he said in the preface:

The use of the Foxglove is getting abroad and it is better the world should derive some instruction, however imperfect, from my experience, than that the lives of men should be hazarded by its unguarded exhibition, or that a medicine of so much efficacy should be condemned and rejected as dangerous and unmanageable.

This book *An Account of the Foxglove* when first published in 1785, was sold, complete with a coloured plate of the foxglove, for only 5/- but, with time, has proved to be one of the classics of medical literature. He considered that one of his important duties was to give a clear warning of the dangers inherent in using digitalis inexpertly. He said:

The Foxglove when given in very large and quickly repeated doses, occasions sickness, vomiting, purging, giddiness, confused vision, objects appearing green or yellow; increased secretion of urine, with frequent motions to part with it, and sometimes inability to retain it; slow pulse, even as slow as 35 in a minute, cold sweats, convulsions, syncope, death.

He stressed that although sufficient of the drug must be given to promote a diuresis, it was not necessary, as he had originally thought, to give it to the point of nausea, in fact he emphasised that nausea, diarrhoea or excessive slowing of the pulse, are signs of over-dosage and should be an indication for stopping the drug.

He considered that the drug should be used whenever there was excess of fluid in the tissues. At that time there was no way of distinguishing between dropsy arising from failure of the heart or kidneys, and therefore Withering must have used it in a certain number of unsuitable cases, not knowing that its action is primarily on the failing heart with its diuretic effect on the kidney secondary to this. Nevertheless, he referred to its powerful action on the motion of the heart and considered that this would prove to be of importance. This concept was really prophetic because although he knew that it slowed the pulse he could not know of its important action in controlling the various disturbances of the heart's rhythm as they were not properly elucidated until the end of the nineteenth century. It is interesting that he differentiated between the wheezing of bronchial asthma, a disease which he surprisingly thought was rare, but rightly said was not helped by digitalis, and wheezing resulting from retention of fluid in the lungs from heart failure and therefore now called cardiac asthma which, as he said, is helped by digitalis.

Withering's book immediately attracted great attention and in the year of publication he was made a Fellow of the Royal Society. Unfortunately, not all physicians shared his enthusiasm for the

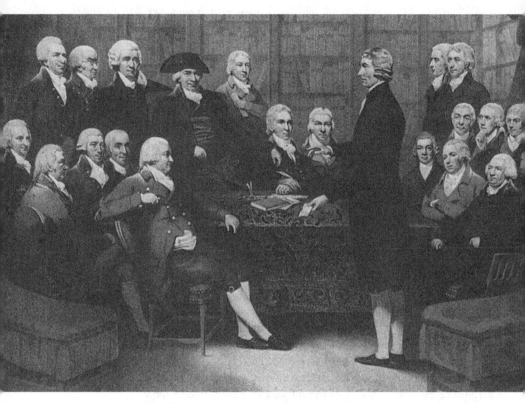

John Coakley Lettsom addressing the Medical Society of London, which he founded in 1773. Membership was at first limited to thirty physicians, thirty surgeons and thirty apothecaries. The figure standing in the background fifth from the left is Edward Jenner (see chapter 6)

drug. Dr John Lettsom, who had the largest and most remunerative practice in London, considered it dangerous as many of his patients died while taking the drug, including Charles James Fox whose dropsy, however, was not due to heart disease but arose from cirrhosis of the liver. Withering, in a letter referring to Lettsom's criticisms, pointed out that no one could compare the London physician's choice of patients with those he considered suitable for the drug, or the manner in which he prescribed it. Regrettably, not only Lettsom but many physicians, ignored Withering's careful instructions and then blamed him when they poisoned their patients. The result of this was that in spite of Withering's efforts to place the administration of digitalis on a proper basis it fell into disrepute for a hundred years until its value was once again recognised in the treatment of heart disorders towards the end of the last century.

It has long been known that drugs helpful in the alleviation of disease are also capable of producing harmful effects and part of the science of medicine is to discover how best to administer them so

that their toxicity is reduced to a minimum. Many promising substances have had to be abandoned because their poisonous effects
have outweighed their benefits but probably from time to time this
has been allowed to happen unnecessarily as either the correct
indication for use, or the best methods of administration, have not
been properly established. For this reason carefully conducted
clinical trials both on animals and, with suitable safeguards, on
patients, are considered essential. The introduction of digitalis long
before this was realised, and its subsequent hazardous progress,
emphasises the wisdom of this modern attitude.

Withering suffered from tuberculosis which finally caused him to
retire from practice in 1783. He continued his botanical studies both
in Great Britain and when he journeyed on the Continent to escape
the English winters. In 1791 his house was ransacked by an angry
mob, at the same time as Priestley's home was burned, because of the
sympathy they had shown towards the French revolutionaries but
fortunately he managed to save most of his precious books and plants
by removing them in wagons camouflaged with straw. When he died,
on 6 October 1799, he was buried in the old church at Edgbaston.

8

Tapping and listening

THE important technique of tapping the chest with the fingers (percussion) and listening to the movements of the heart and lungs with a stethoscope (auscultation) are so commonly performed by physicians as to be familiar to everyone. At times, because they appear to be conducted in a manner somewhat reminiscent of a ceremonial ritual, they have perhaps contributed an aura of mystique to physical examination. As they are seemingly straightforward procedures, it might be assumed that they have been in use from time immemorial whereas, in fact, they are relatively recent skills. Percussion was first applied to the practice of medicine in the middle of the eighteenth century and auscultation not until the early part of the nineteenth century.

Joseph Leopold Auenbrugger (1722–1809) the son of an innkeeper who lived in Gratz in Austria was the first physician to gain information from tapping with his fingers on his patients' chests. After completing his medical studies at the University of Vienna he obtained an appointment, in 1751, as assistant physician to the Spanish Military Hospital in that city. It was in 1754 that he first noted that percussion over different parts of the chest wall produces sounds of varying pitch depending on the type of structure underneath. Undoubtedly he gained the idea from his boyhood when he had seen the sides of barrels being tapped to discover how much wine they contained, for in his work on percussion he remarked that casks, as long as they are empty, are uniformly resonant, but when filled lose this property. It is surprising that no physician before him had thought to apply the method to diagnosis, as undoubtedly it had been practised for centuries, not only in the examination of barrels but also for many other purposes, including the testing of walls to see whether they were solid or covered hiding places. The procedure must have appeared attractive to him because he had a well developed musical ear which enabled him, amongst other achievements, to write the libretto for the opera *The Chimney Sweep*.

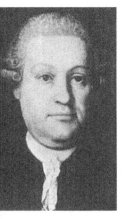

Joseph Leopold Auenbrugger (1722–1809)

After he had practised this technique for seven years, he published his observations in 1761 in the ninety-five-page book, *Inventum Novum ex Percussione Thoracis Humani Ut Signo Abstrusos Interni Pectoris Morbos Detegendi* (New invention, by means of percussing the human chest, as a sign of detecting obscure diseases in the interior of the chest). He felt obliged to publish his findings because he was certain that they would prove helpful to his colleagues, but he did not relish the publicity because, like Harvey, when he published *De motu cordis*, he realised that human nature was such that his motives for publication might well be misinterpreted and his reputation harmed. In his preface therefore he states:

In making public my discoveries respecting this matter, I have been actuated neither by an itch for writing, nor a fondness for speculation, but by the desire of submitting to my brethren the fruits of seven years observation and reflection. In doing so, I have not been unconscious of the dangers I must encounter; since it has always been the fate of those who have illustrated or improved the arts and sciences by their discoveries, to be beset by envy, malice, hatred, detraction and calumny.

Undeterred by such considerations he says,

what I have written I have proved again and again by the testimony of my own senses, and amid laborious and tedious exertions—still guarding, on all occasions, against the seductive influence of self love.

His method of percussion was to strike the chest wall with the tips of the extended fingers: he found that the note produced was better if elicited either with the shirt drawn tightly over the chest or with the physician's hand covered with a leather glove. Since his time the technique has undergone various modifications and it is now common practice to lay one hand flat on the bare chest and to strike the back of its middle finger with the tip of the middle finger of the other hand. Auenbrugger found that the vibration set up on percussion of the chest wall overlying healthy lungs by his method gave a resonant note which he likened to 'the stifled sound of a drum covered with a thick woollen cloth or other envelope'. By systematic percussion over all areas of the chest he was able to define the boundaries of the lungs; also he observed that, because of diminished resonance, the percussion note is impaired over the heart and any part of the lungs rendered airless by disease. Again, when the pleural cavity surrounding the lungs or the pericardial sac around the heart becomes filled with fluid, the sound produced by percussion is so muffled as to produce a completely dull note. He was well aware that there were certain practical difficulties in the interpretation of these sounds, including the variations produced by differing degrees of thickness of the chest wall, depending on the amount of fat or thickness of muscle which may be present. Although radiological examination, available since the end of the last century, has made the assessment of respiratory and cardiac disease more accurate, nevertheless percussion is still a useful procedure and certainly in Auenbrugger's time its importance should immediately have been recognised. Unfortunately this was not so, even Baron van Swieten, Professor of Medicine at Vienna University whom Auenbrugger had held in the highest respect since his student days, ignored the discovery so that his treatise published in 1764 on fluid around the lungs in pulmonary tuberculosis made no mention of percussion.

The year after Auenbrugger published his book, he was dismissed from the Spanish Military Hospital where he was by that time the chief physician, and subsequently devoted himself entirely to private practice. The poor reception of his book does not seem to have embittered him, possibly because he had a happy marriage, his private practice prospered and he was popular at the Court of Vienna where he developed a close friendship with the Empress Maria Theresa and was ennobled by the Emperor Joseph II with the title 'Edler von Auenbrugg' in 1784.

Fortunately, Maximilian Stoll, one of the foremost physicians in Vienna at that time, adopted the art of percussion and taught the technique to his students from 1776–84 as well as describing the method in certain of his publications. The *Inventum Novum* was translated into French by Rozière of Montpellier in 1770 but, in spite of there being two editions of this translation, the method still did not come into general use until popularised by the famous French clinician Jean Nicolas Corvisart.

Corvisart (1755–1821), born in the tiny French village of Dricourt, was sent at an early age to live with his uncle, a parish priest at Vimille. During his childhood he appears to have shown no aptitude for learning but on the contrary was said to be lazy, mischievous and quarrelsome. Nevertheless, matriculating at the age of thirteen, he then started training as a lawyer. While studying for the bar, he visited many hospitals in Paris which led him to decide that he would rather train to be a doctor. As this led to a family row and his expulsion from home he took a resident post at the famous Hôtel-Dieu in Paris so as to have the opportunity to study medicine whilst being assured of his board and lodging. He proved to be an outstanding student and after qualification soon obtained important hospital posts. In 1788 he was appointed physician to the Charité Hospital and when, in 1795, the Medical School was established there, he was chosen to occupy the chair of medicine. In 1797 he became Professor of Medicine at the Collège de France and in 1799 a physician to the Government.

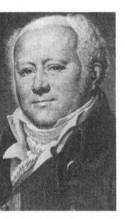

Jean Nicolas Corvisart (1755–1821)

Foremost among his patients and personal friends was Napoleon

Bonaparte who in 1798 presented him with a large carved mahogany chair. This he placed in his consulting room and it is still a much prized and highly valued antique in the possession of the Corvisart family. In 1804 he received the official appointment of Personal Physician to the Emperor. It seems that they greatly enjoyed each other's company and several accounts of conversations between them have been recorded. On one occasion, when the Emperor, who had a constant fear of being poisoned, was rolling on the ground with nothing more wrong with him than a mild attack of indigestion, Corvisart is said to have admonished him by exclaiming, 'Get up! What would be said if the Master of the World were seen thus crushed by fear?' When Napoleon's son was born in 1811 Corvisart is reported to have said:

'Sire, this child should fulfil your last wish, consider from what a position you have arisen in less than ten years: Lieutenant, Captain, Brigadier-General, General in Chief, First Consul, Emperor, Spouse of an Austrian Archduchess, and the father of a male child. You have reached the summit of the wheel of fortune and of great renown. Stop Sire, or Destiny may desert you and then nothing remains but downfall and disaster.'

'Well,' replied the Emperor, 'that was such a speech as one would expect from a native of the Champagne.'

Corvisart's many distinguished women patients included the Empress Josephine, the Empress Marie-Louise, the Queen of Holland, the Queen of Spain and Napoleon's sister, Pauline.

In addition to his private practice he contributed much to the teaching of medicine and, being particularly interested in diseases of the heart, presented many of his original observations in his book *Essai sur les maladies du cœur et des gros vaisseaux* published in 1806. Also, realising the importance of work done in other countries, he translated into French books written in many languages, including those of Max Stoll.

It was from a study of Stoll's writings and not from Rozière's French translation of Auenbrugger's book that Corvisart first learned of percussion. As soon as he read it he immediately recognised its importance but it was not until he had practised the method for twenty years that, in 1808, a year before Auenbrugger's death, he published his translation of the *Inventum Novum* with additional commentaries based on his own experience. Although Corvisart made it clear that it was Auenbrugger who deserved all the credit for the discovery, there is no doubt that the widespread acceptance of percussion was entirely due to the French physician's prestige and authority.

Napoleon continued to have the benefit of Corvisart's friendship and professional advice until soon after the Battle of Waterloo, when

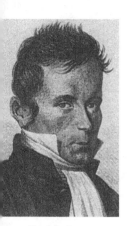

*René Laënnec
(1781–1826)*

his physician was forced to retire from the practice of medicine following a stroke. Both men died in 1821, the Emperor from cancer on 5 May, the physician from a further stroke on 15 September.

One of the many students privileged to be taught by Corvisart was René Théophile Hyacinthe Laënnec (1781–1826) and it was he who, in a comparatively short life, became himself a great teacher and the inventor of the stethoscope. He was born of a tuberculous mother at Quimper in Lower Brittany. His mother died a few years later following childbirth and as his father, an impecunious lawyer, found the rearing of René and his brother too much for him he sent them to live with their uncle Michel, the rector of a parish in Elliant. This cleric, sensing the onset of the French Revolution, decided, in 1788, to move to England, so the two boys went to their other and more famous uncle, Guillaume-François Laënnec. This uncle had many cultural interests, in addition to being the Professor of Medicine at the University of Nantes. He encouraged his nephew in the pursuit of a broad comprehensive education and there is no doubt that René was very happy in his home in spite of the bitter turmoil into which the country had been plunged. The family was not spared the horror of the Revolution, because a guillotine stood in the square outside their house and the boys must have seen many decapitations, in addition to living through the harrowing experience of their uncle being imprisoned for six weeks under suspicion of being out of sympathy with the government.

In 1795, at the early age of fourteen and a half, Laënnec began the study of medicine at L'Hôtel-Dieu at Nantes where his uncle was in charge of one hundred of the beds, most of them occupied by sailors suffering from tropical diseases. After five years his uncle advised him to move to Paris where, as a student at L'École de Médicine, he was taught by several famous men including Corvisart who, of all his teachers, had the greatest influence on his career.

As a student Laënnec proved his abilities as an original observer and in 1802 published an account of the appearances of a severely damaged mitral valve at post-mortem examination and in 1804, shortly before he graduated, delivered an important lecture showing that the wasting disease up to then known as pthisis, was in reality pulmonary tuberculosis. Eight years later he was appointed physician to the Beaujon Hospital where he became especially interested in diseases of the chest and used the technique of percussion taught him by Corvisart. In 1816 he became a physician at the Necker Hospital and it was there, during the first year of his appointment, that he developed the art of auscultation.

Auscultation, a word derived from the Latin *auscultatio* and the French *auscultari*—listen to—is applied mainly to the act of listening to sounds arising in the body from movements within the heart, blood vessels, lungs or intestines. The direct application of the ear to the chest wall to listen to the lungs must have been practised in ancient Greece because the characteristic splash heard when fluid and air occupy the pleural space surrounding the lungs is described in Hippocratic writings about 400 B.C. There was no mention however of heart sounds until 1616, when Harvey, in his Lumleian lecture (now the property of the British Museum) wrote, 'It is plain from the structure of the heart that the blood is passed continuously through the lungs to the aorta as by the two clacks of a water bellows to raise water'. 'Clack', an onamatopoeic term also used in Harvey's time to describe a pump valve, suggests that he was using the word in order to describe sounds which he correctly surmised were of valvular origin. Others found them difficult to hear, for Aurelius Parisanus wrote scathingly in 1647, 'nor we, poor deafs, nor any other doctor in Venice can hear them, but happy is he who can hear them in London'. Robert Hooke the physicist, however, had no such difficulty and clearly foresaw the diagnostic value of auscultation when about the same time he wrote:

I have been able to hear very plainly the beating of a man's heart ... who knows, I say, but that it may be possible to discover the motions of the internal parts of bodies ... by the sound they make, that one may discover the works performed in the several offices and shops of a man's body and thereby discover what instrument or engine is out of order.

The usefulness of the method in diagnosis was confirmed when James Douglas of St Bartholomew's Hospital, London, reported in 1715 a case where the noise in a patient's chest from the disordered action of his heart was so loud that it could not only be detected when the ear was placed to the chest, but could on occasions be readily heard at some distance from the bedside. William Hunter, the London surgeon, in 1757 described a patient in whom he had heard a noise caused by blood passing through an abnormal communication between an artery and vein (arteriovenous fistula). He compared the noise to that produced by air passing through a small opening or to the sound of the letter 'r' spoken in a prolonged whisper. An arteriovenous fistula may occur when there is injury to an artery and vein lying close together. This was not an uncommon occurrence in the days of frequent sword fights and Joseph Hodgson, a Birmingham surgeon, described in 1815 a patient who, following a sword wound, developed a noise in the upper part of the thigh which was so loud as to be audible at a distance of three or four inches.

The first textbook on cardiology in the English language was written by Allan Burns of Glasgow in 1809 and in this he mentions sounds heard on listening to the heart. An interesting reference to direct auscultation was also given by F. J. Double of Paris when, in 1817, he described an occasion when his mother, sadly bidding him farewell, pulled his head to her bosom as she wept. He says he was struck by the distinct manner in which he heard the beating of her heart and the convulsive sobs in her breathing. The sounds of the foetal heart heard when an ear is placed on the abdomen of a pregnant woman were demonstrated by François Mayor, a surgeon in Geneva, to some of his colleagues in 1818.

It is obvious therefore that by the early part of the nineteenth century many people were using direct auscultation and finding it helpful as a diagnostic procedure. It is, therefore, of much interest to learn that Corvisart, one of the foremost cardiologists of that time, thought little of it. He paid great attention to the general appearance of his patients and looked carefully for normal and abnormal pulsations in the heart and great vessels. Further, he used his hands, not only for percussion but for feeling the movement of the heart and the pulse at the wrist. He described how sometimes, when the mitral valve is damaged by disease so that it ceases to open properly, vibrations are set up which may be felt by placing a hand flat on the chest. He called the sensation produced by these vibrations a *bruissement*, a word also used in French to describe the buzzing of bees, the rustling of leaves or the murmuring of a brook. He was aware that it was possible to hear noises arising in the heart for, in his book, he refers to the assertion made by some people that when the noises are particularly loud they may be heard standing a short distance from the patient's bed. Contemptuously he remarked, 'I have never had an opportunity, I repeat it, of ascertaining these unquestionably rare observations; I have barely heard these sounds by applying my ear close to the patient's thorax'.

His disregard for auscultation is evident from his case reports and also from the fact that Laënnec stated that he had never, on any occasion, seen the professor apply his ear to the chest. Laënnec said it was Gaspard-Laurent Bayle who first introduced him to the technique when they were studying cases together on Corvisart's wards. Laënnec was quick to appreciate its usefulness but considered there were certain important factors which limited its use, for he said, '... as inconvenient for the physician as for the patient, distaste alone renders it almost impracticable in the hospital, it cannot even be proposed to most women and in most of them the volume of the breasts is a physical obstacle to its use'. The manner in which he discovered how these difficulties might be overcome is graphically described, together with other important observations made over several years, in his famous book *Traité de l'auscultation médiate* which first appeared in 1819:

In 1816, I was consulted by a young woman labouring under general symptoms of diseased heart, and in whose case percussion and the application of the hand were of little avail on account of the great degree of fatness. The other method just mentioned being rendered inadmissible by the age and sex of the patient, I happened to recollect a simple and well-known fact in acoustics, and fancied at the same time, that it might be turned to some use on the present occasion. The fact I allude to is the augmented impression of sound when conveyed through certain solid bodies, as when we hear the scratch of a pin at one end of a piece of wood, on applying our ear to the other. Immediately, on this suggestion, I rolled a quire of paper into a sort of cylinder and applied one end of it to the region of the heart and the other to my ear and was not a little surprised and pleased, to find that I could thereby perceive the action of the heart in a manner much more clear and distinct than I had ever been able to do by the immediate application of the ear. From this moment I imagined that the circumstance might furnish means for enabling us to ascertain the character not only of the action of the heart, but of every species of sound produced by the motion of all the thoracic viscera.

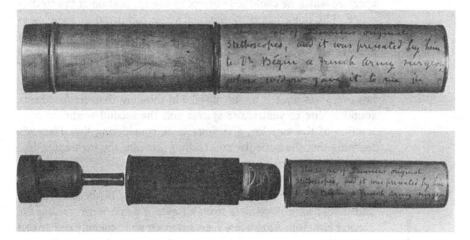

An original Laënnec stethoscope. The lower illustration shows how the parts fit together

The acoustic principle underlying this invention was well known to Leonardo da Vinci who observed that ships at a distance could readily be heard by placing one end of an oar in the water and applying the ear to the other end, but it is most unlikely that Leonardo's writings were known to Laënnec. As soon as Laënnec found how easily he could hear the heart sounds with the aid of the quire of paper he replaced it by a wooden cylinder which, as one of his hobbies was wood turning, he readily made on his own lathe. The cylinder had a hole three inches in diameter bored down the centre, with one end hollowed out in the shape of a funnel. This instrument, first called by him 'the cylinder', soon became known as a stethoscope, a word derived from the Greek 'stethos' (chest). He used the instrument for three years before publishing his observations with it and during that time conscientiously correlated the sounds he had heard in life with the pathological changes found after death. His main interest was in diseases of the lungs and he wrote an important book on this subject, but he also made valuable observations on disorders of the heart and, by the use of the stethoscope, was able to add to knowledge already obtained by Corvisart. He confirmed his professor's teaching that a peculiar sensation may be felt on placing a hand on the chest wall over a stenosed* valve and, likening it to the purring of a cat, called it *frémissement cataire*. He realised that it is only present when the narrowing of the valve orifice is severe, and had only encountered the sign in three cases of mitral valve stenosis† by the time he wrote his book on auscultation. Far more common, in his experience, were lesser degrees of contraction of the valve aperture which he could only detect by the application of the stethoscope. The noise heard by this means he compared in some cases with the rasping of a file on wood (*bruit de râpe*) and in others to a bellows sharply compressed (*bruit de soufflet*). A study of these noises, known in the English language as murmurs, has proved of the greatest value in diagnosis. Laënnec's interpretation of them, however, was limited by his mistake in thinking that the first heart sound is due to ventricular systole and the second sound to contraction of the auricles; a curious error considering that Harvey's teaching that the auricular contraction precedes the ventricular had long been accepted.

His colleagues in France at first treated his discovery with indifference but the first edition of 3,500 copies of his book soon sold and before long physicians from all over Europe were visiting the Necker Hospital. After a few years his merit was generally recognised so that he was appointed Professor of Medicine in the Collège de France in 1822 and at the same time became a member of the Academy of Medicine of France; two years later he was made a Knight of the Legion of Honour.

Unfortunately, Laënnec suffered from pulmonary tuberculosis, one of the diseases to which he contributed such important knowledge. His health was so poor when he prepared his book on auscultation that later he said he knew that the effort entailed in writing it might kill him but considered the contents would be far more valuable than the life of a man. He in fact became so ill, once his book was published, that immediately afterwards he had to give up

---

*From Greek 'stenos'—narrow.
†Valve stenosis—narrowing of valve orifice by disease process.

work for a short time to recuperate in his native Brittany. A year later he was forced to return there and on that occasion had to stay for two years. After his health had sufficiently recovered he returned to Paris to take up practice again and began a revision of his book. By 1826, however, his health had once more seriously deteriorated and he had to retire to Brittany where he died on 13 August at the age of forty-five. Fortunately he lived long enough to have the satisfaction of seeing the use of the stethoscope widely accepted and its worth appreciated.

The first English edition of Laënnec's book, published in 1821, was a poor translation by Sir John Forbes but the invention created such interest in England that the London *Times* of 19 September 1824, commented:

A wonderful instrument called the stethoscope ... is now in complete vogue in Paris. It is merely a hollow wooden tube (a common flute with the holes stopped and the top open would do just as well). One end is applied to the breast of the patient the other to the ear of the physician and according to different sounds harsh, hollow, soft, loud, etc. he judges of the state of the disease. It is quite a fashion, if a person complains of cough, to have recourse to the miraculous tube which however cannot effect a cure but should you unfortunately perceive in the countenance of the doctor that he fancies certain symptoms exist it is very likely that a nervous person might become seriously indisposed and convert the supposition into reality.

Auscultation was soon widely practised in the English-speaking world; in London it was enthusiastically taught by Charles J. B. Williams at the Brompton Hospital, by James Hope at St George's Hospital, and by Thomas Hodgkin at Guy's Hospital. And in Ireland, by the Dublin physicians William Stokes, Robert Adams, Robert Graves and Sir Dominic Corrigan; Stokes, at the age of twenty-one, publishing a small book on auscultation in 1825, the year he qualified. In America the attention of physicians was directed to auscultation by Sir John Forbes's translation of Laënnec's *Treatise on Diseases of the Chest* published in Philadelphia in 1823.

Improvements in the design of Laënnec's instrument were gradually introduced, Pierre-Adolphe Piorry made the instrument-less clumsy by reducing its diameter to that of a finger and also he incorporated a trumpet chest-piece and modified the ear-piece. His model was in use in France for the next eighty years. Rigid stethoscopes were made of a variety of materials including deal, which was the favourite, ebony, metal and even glass. The length was variable, some people using specially long ones, based on the distance it was considered fleas could jump! The next advance was the introduction of a flexible stethoscope with tubing, originally made of caoutchouc (unvulcanised rubber). One authority considered this type to be far

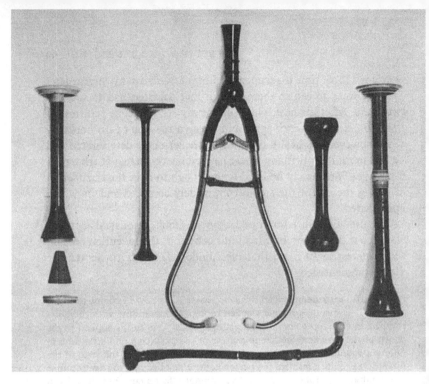

Some mid-nineteenth-century stethoscopes

superior as the physician's head did not have to be over the chest of the sick person and because the tubing could be readily lengthened, so avoiding 'too close proximity to contagious cases and the miserably wretched' and enabling it to be used 'in the highest ranks of society without offending fastidious delicacy'.

The introduction by Charles Goodyear, in 1844, of vulcanised rubber, led to a great improvement in the quality of the flexible stethoscope but for several years it continued to consist of only a single tube. The first binaural model, a precursor of the type in use today, was invented by George P. Cammann in America in 1852. It was soon in regular use in England, but in France, the country of birth of the stethoscope, doctors were peculiarly conservative so that even in the early part of this century many of them still auscultated by applying the ear direct to a thin handkerchief placed on the patient's chest, and the binaural stethoscope was not introduced there until about 1910.

Diagnosis in recent years has been greatly assisted by the introduction of much complex scientific machinery but the place of auscultation with the stethoscope is still as important as ever in the assessment of cardiac disorders. Our present knowledge of the subject has not been easily acquired, but has depended on the work of numerous physicians from the beginning of the nineteenth century to the present day.

9

The use and misuse of the stethoscope

THE invention of the stethoscope was to lead to a revolutionary improvement in the diagnosis of the various disorders which affect the heart and lungs; first, however, the necessary skill in the correct interpretation of the numerous and complex sounds which arise from these organs had to be acquired. This did not prove easy and initially, as might be expected, many mistakes were made. But when it is considered how difficult at times it is even today to arrive at a correct diagnosis, when information gained from auscultation may be supplemented by that obtained from other more sophisticated diagnostic procedures such as radiology and electrocardiography, the formidable task which faced the physicians at the beginning of the nineteenth century may readily be appreciated.

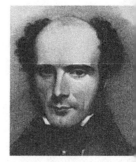

James Hope (1801–41)

One of the pioneers of auscultation in England was James Hope (1801–41). Hope, born in Stockport, Cheshire, son of a wealthy merchant, wanted, when he left Macclesfield Grammar School at the age of eighteen, to become a lawyer. His ambition was however thwarted by the Manchester Riots in 1819 which led him to enlist in the Yeomanry Lancers. On demobilisation about twelve months later he decided, on the advice of his father, to study medicine and it was for this pupose that he went to Edinburgh. It is said that he found the practical work in the Anatomy Department most distasteful and always dissected wearing a pair of gloves. He seems quickly to have overcome such squeamishness and to have been an able student for, in his second year, he was invited to join the Royal Medical Society of Edinburgh to which learned society he presented a paper on the heart. It was the enthusiastic manner in which this was received that decided him to make a special study of disorders of this organ. After qualification he served as a house physician and house surgeon at the Edinburgh Royal Infirmary. By the end of this period he had completed a thesis for his doctorate of medicine in which he proved that it was possible to diagnose the presence of an abnormal dilatation or aneurysm of the aorta during the life of a patient, a task which Laënnec had previously said was not possible.

Hope, deciding that he wanted to practise as a doctor in London next went to St Bartholomew's Hospital in 1826 where he spent a year preparing himself for the examination of the Royal College of Surgeons of England. Following a further year of study on the Continent he returned to London where he started as a practitioner whilst continuing the study of medicine at St George's Hospital. At that time the physicians there had a strong prejudice against the use of the stethoscope but Hope was not deterred by this and, although only attending the hospital as a student, made many original observations from auscultation of patients with diseased hearts. At the same time he carried out important experiments on donkeys in order to determine the significance of the various sounds heard both in health and disease. His methods were somewhat unfortunate because they involved the performance of major surgery on these animals after having hit them on the head to render them unconscious, or after the administration of the poison woorara, now better known as curare. In his account of the first series of experiments, published in the *London Medical Gazette* in 1830, he says:

An ass of which the pulse and impulse were 48 per minute, was instantaneously deprived of sensation and motion by a smart blow on the head. The trachea was opened, a large bellows-pipe introduced and artificial respiration maintained; while at the same time the left ribs were sawn through near the sternum and forcibly bent back and broken so as widely and completely to expose the heart immediately behind the left shoulder: this was accomplished in less than five minutes...

In his description of a further series of experiments published in his book of 1839 he says:

a large ass, aged eight or nine, with a pulse of 50 was employed. The jugular vein having been denuded ... a small incision was made in the vessel just sufficient to admit an ounce syringe charged with a solution of 2 grains of woorara in an ounce of water. This being injected ... respiration instantly began to fail and in less than a minute had nearly ceased, and in a minute wholly. The trachea was then opened, a bellows-pipe introduced and artificial respiration established.

The action of curare is to paralyse all the muscles of the body under voluntary control including those of the chest wall, and it was for this reason that his animals had to be artificially ventilated, but as the drug has no effect on the sensory part of the nervous system the animals would have been conscious of all painful stimuli. Hope, who was a humane man, possibly was not aware of this and no doubt was influenced in his choice of method by the great interest being shown in the drug at that time; Sir Benjamin Brodie, a surgeon at St George's Hospital, who provided the curare for Hope's experiments, had smeared woorara paste on wounds of guinea pigs in 1811 and noted that death could be delayed by inflating the lungs through a tube introduced into the trachea. Also the traveller, Charles Waterton, in his *Wanderings in South America* gave an account of his search for woorara used by the natives there as an arrow poison. A revised edition of this book was published in 1828, the year Hope started work in London. In this Waterton discusses the suggestion that a person poisoned by this substance might be revived by inflating the lungs but obviously he didn't think much of the idea for he comments, 'It may be so; but this is a difficult and tedious mode of cure.' Nevertheless, he later put the method to the test when, having poisoned a donkey with the substance, he incised the windpipe and inflated the lungs with a pair of bellows for two hours. This procedure saved the donkey's life and, in recompense for its sufferings, it was named Wouralia and allowed to live in idleness for the next twenty-five years.

Hope derived far more information from his experiments. With the heart exposed he was able to correlate the sounds heard on auscultation with the movements of the organ. By this means he was able to demonstrate that the first heart sound and the second heart sound mark the beginning and the end of each ventricular contraction and that the second sound is produced by the abrupt closure of the aortic and pulmonary valves.

Hope's experiments were carried out in the presence of many witnesses, the reason for this being that as there was no method of recording the results it was essential to have the confirmation of as many observers as possible. One influential participant in these experiments was the Brompton Hospital physician, Charles J. B. Williams, and unfortunately much bitterness developed between the two men as the result of arguments over the cause of the first sound. Williams believed, and stated in the third edition of his book published in 1835, that it was due to the muscular contraction of the heart's ventricles. Hope, on the other hand, considered the first sound to be valvular as well as muscular in origin. He was nearer to the truth for it is now accepted that it is produced by the closure of the mitral and tricuspid valves.

As freely acknowledged by Williams, it was Hope who was in the main responsible for the correct interpretation of many of the murmurs heard in heart disease. He was much helped in this by his experiments on donkeys as, for example, when on one occasion he purposely damaged the pulmonary valve and found that the murmur produced was similar to that heard when blood regurgitates through an incompetent aortic valve.

A very clear description of Hope's animal experiments and observations on over a thousand patients is given in the third edition

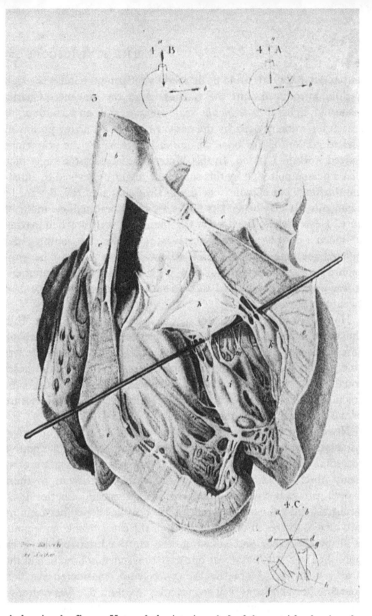

A drawing by James Hope of the interior of the left ventricle showing the chordae tendinae (with a rod behind them) attached to the undersurface of the mitral valve

of his treatise on diseases of the heart published in 1839. This book, beautifully illustrated with his own drawings, is a masterpiece and was far in advance of its time.

Also in 1839 he was appointed a full physician at St George's Hospital, having been an assistant physician there for the previous five years. Unfortunately, his health had been failing because of pulmonary tuberculosis, a disease which also affected many of his brothers and sisters, and it was this which caused his death in May 1841, at the age of forty.

A study of the different kinds of murmur soon showed that it is possible to distinguish between two separate types of valve damage. One, where the cusps of a valve, because of inflammatory or degenerative disease, become thickened and stiff so that they do not open properly, is known as valve stenosis. The second where the cusps of a valve, eroded and partially destroyed by disease, do not fit tightly when the valve closes, thus allowing regurgitation of blood, is known as valve incompetence. This term, although widely used, is unsatisfactory, as a stenosed valve is also incompetent. The disorder is therefore better referred to as valve regurgitation. Sometimes a valve may show evidence of both stenosis and regurgitation. The two valves most commonly affected in this way by acquired disease are the mitral valve (situated between the left atrium and left ventricle) and the aortic valve (situated at the mouth of the aorta where it arises from the left ventricle). The principal disease which affects the mitral valve is rheumatic fever. The aortic valve may also be damaged by this disease as well as by degenerative arterio-sclerotic changes; and in the past was not uncommonly affected by syphilis, but this has now become rare since the introduction of penicillin for the treatment of this infection.

James Hope, in the 1839 edition of his book, made a clear distinction between the signs of mitral valve incompetence and stenosis. He pointed out that when the valve, because of damage to the cusps, is permanently open, so as to allow regurgitation of blood into the left auricle when the left ventricle contracts, there is a rough rasping or smooth bellows type of murmur during the interval between the first and second heart sounds. He described it as being low in key, more or less like whispering 'who', and heard particularly well over the apex of the heart (the point where the normal heart beat is felt, just below the left nipple); sometimes it is so loud at this site as to completely drown the first sound and is frequently accompanied by a palpable purring tremor. The murmur of mitral stenosis, he said, is heard in the same situation as the murmur of mitral incompetence but is different in its timing, being heard during the interval between the second and the first heart sounds and usually on a rather lower key than a whispered 'who'. Erroneously he said that the murmur of mitral stenosis is never accompanied by a purring tremor felt with the hand and he also failed to make it clear that the typical murmur of mitral stenosis comes just before the first sound, the so-called pre-systolic murmur. It was Sulpice Antoine Fauvel who first used this term in 1843 when he described the intense rasping murmur (*bruit de râpe*) preceding the first sound in five cases of mitral stenosis.

Hope also recognised many of the signs of aortic stenosis and aortic incompetence but credit for the best description of the latter must be given to the Irish physician, Sir Dominic John Corrigan whose paper on the subject was first published in 1832.

Corrigan (1802–80) was born in Dublin, the son of a successful farmer. His education at the Catholic College of St Patrick at Maynooth was followed by an apprenticeship to Dr O'Kelly, physician to the College. O'Kelly was so impressed with the lad that he persuaded his father to send him to Edinburgh University to study medicine. While there he was a contemporary of William Stokes, another Irishman destined to make important contributions to our knowledge of heart disease. Soon after graduation in 1825 Corrigan settled in Dublin. His particular interest in cardiology became evident when in 1829 he published a paper in the *Lancet* entitled 'An Aneurysm of the Aorta'.* This was of importance at the time as it emphasised the value of the stethoscope in the diagnosis of heart disease and was followed two months later by two papers in the same journal in which he discussed Laënnec's conception of the *bruit de soufflet* and *frémissement cataire*. Laënnec had taught that these sometimes resulted from spasm of the arteries but Corrigan correctly put forward an explanation based on the flow properties of liquids.

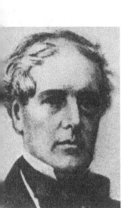

Sir Dominic Corrigan (1802–80)

In 1830 he was appointed physician to the Jervis Street Hospital where, although he had only six beds he quickly established a reputation as a physician, pathologist and teacher. His most famous paper, and the one on which his immortality as a cardiologist rests, was published in the *Edinburgh Medical Journal* in 1832, when he was aged thirty, under the title 'On Permanent Patency of the Mouth of the Aorta, or Inadequacy of the Aortic Valves' in which he discusses the symptoms, signs, causes and treatment of aortic valve incompetence.

His honest belief that he was the first to describe this disorder was violently opposed by James Hope, who claimed that he had first done so in 1825 and that he had followed this in 1831 with a description of the typical jerky type of pulse found in this condition. Both were wrong for attention had first been drawn to it by William Cowper in 1705 in the *Philosophical Transactions of the Royal Society*; Raymond Vieussens, in 1715, also gave a strikingly accurate account of a case of mitral stenosis and a case of aortic incompetence, both with autopsy confirmation. Vieussens knew nothing of course about murmurs, but his patient with mitral stenosis he described as having lips the colour of lead and a pulse 'very small, feeble and absolutely uneven', whilst his patient with aortic incompetence he described as

*Aneurysm—the ballooning of part of an artery from the Greek *aneursma*.

pale and having a pulse 'very full, very fast, hard, uneven and so strong that the arteries of both arms struck the ends of my fingers like a cord which had been tightly stretched and then violently shaken'; an excellent description of these two very different types of pulse. Thomas Hodgkin, the Quaker physician at Guy's Hospital, also gave an account of aortic valve incompetence three years before Corrigan's classic paper.

None of these however compares with the completeness of the picture presented by Corrigan, including his description of the characteristic collapsing pulse since when often referred to as Corrigan's pulse, as well as his reference to the marked pulsation of the arteries in the neck and arms, also the characteristic murmur heard over the aortic area and main arteries of the neck and arms when the ventricles are in diastole. He pointed out that when the aortic valve is so grossly damaged as to allow a large amount of blood to regurgitate into the left ventricle, a double murmur may be heard over the ascending aorta; the first part he thought was produced by blood rushing up the aorta and the second part by it running back into the ventricle. This to and fro type of murmur, as it is now often called, has since been recognised to be a common finding with aortic valve incompetence.

He was not certain of the causes of aortic incompetence. In only one of his eleven cases was there a clear past history of rheumatic fever, now known to be one of the principal underlying diseases. Also, he had no knowledge of the part that syphilis plays in destroying the aortic valve although this infection must have been a common cause at that time. He does however mention that this type of valve damage is not infrequently associated with an abnormal dilatation or aneurysm of the aorta, a condition which long before his time was suspected of being of syphilitic origin. It was not however until the causative organism of syphilis had been identified by Schaudinn in 1905 that its effects on the aortic valve could be proved.

It is thus clear that during the first half of the nineteenth century many physicians developed considerable skill in the use of the stethoscope. With time they began to appreciate that certain murmurs heard during ventricular systole are not caused by heart disease but may arise in other conditions such as anaemia, or at times in normal people. Auscultation therefore brought with it serious responsibilities as the various types of murmur had to be distinguished and appropriate advice given accordingly. Some of the difficulties in the early days were admirably discussed by the American physician, Austin Flint. Flint, who came of a family with a strong medical tradition, was appointed Professor of Medicine at Bellevue Hospital, New York, in 1859, an appointment he held until

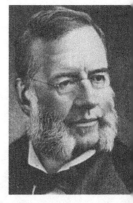

Austin Flint (1812–86)

his death from a cerebral haemorrhage in 1886. In his paper 'On Cardiac Murmurs' in 1862 he pointed out that prior to the discovery of the stethoscope, heart disease was only diagnosed at a very late stage, when symptoms of shortness of breath, palpitations and dropsy were well established and death never long delayed. This led to a deep-rooted conviction that heart disease is always of extreme seriousness so when the stethoscope was invented all patients found to have murmurs, regardless of the cause, including those with little or no disturbance of their health, were given a grave prognosis and subjected to intensive treatment expressly designed to weaken and debilitate them. No wonder that Flint said, '... so long as the notions with regard to treatment of cardiac affections prevailed, an early diagnosis, instead of being desirable, was a serious disadvantage and truly fortunate were they who kept aloof from the stethoscope of the auscultator'.

In his paper he discusses personal experiences which led him to appreciate the folly of the current belief that all patients with heart murmurs have an equally bad outlook. He describes how he informed the mother of one eleven-year-old girl with a very loud murmur and enlargement of the heart that her daughter would soon be dead, only to find the patient alive thirteen years later. Also, how having confidently predicted an early death for a man found to have a loud murmur and enlarged heart at a routine life assurance examination, discovered he was alive and very active twenty years later. His account of the case history of a fellow medical practitioner illustrates how anxiety engendered in an otherwise fit man by failure to distinguish between an innocent and serious type of murmur may lead to much unnecessary ill-health. This unfortunate doctor, having been informed by a colleague that he had a murmur and being of an anxious and introspective temperament, quickly developed distressing symptoms. Flint says that by the time he was consulted for a second opinion the man's apprehension had led him to become severely incapacitated although examination revealed only a faint murmur from minimal damage of one valve and another murmur which, although loud when the heart rate was rapid, disappeared when the patient rested. This, as Flint says, was obviously an entirely innocent type of murmur of no significance and only caused concern at the first examination because the doctor was unwise enough to examine the patient immediately after the exertion of climbing a flight of stairs. Such errors of judgment unfortunately continued to be common for the rest of the nineteenth century, as may be learned from the writings of Sir James Mackenzie. Mackenzie, whose life will be fully discussed later, was an outstanding person who, as a result of his many original contributions to our knowledge of heart disease whilst in general practice, gained for himself such an international reputation that eventually he became head of the Cardiology Department at the London Hospital in the early part of this century. Perhaps best known for his ingenious use of the polygraph which enabled him to recognise the different disorders of heart rhythm and to separate the dangerous ones from those which may safely be ignored, as a young man he also realised the importance of distinguishing between the various types of murmur. This he did by first making an accurate analysis of the sounds and then by following the progress of his patients over a long period. From this study during forty years of general practice, he learned not only how to distinguish innocent from serious types of murmur but also came to realise that the outlook for patients with the latter varies widely and depends to a large extent on the capacity of the heart muscle to respond to effort. This he found could best be assessed by reference to the two cardinal symptoms of chest pain and shortness of breath. He taught, for instance, that when a young woman with mitral stenosis enquires whether it is safe for her to undergo the stress of pregnancy, the advice given should depend not so much on information derived from examination with the stethoscope as it should from the patient's own assessment as to whether or not there has been any recent and unusual shortness of breath on exertion. He realised that not only adults but also children are the best judge of their own capabilities and taught parents that it is best to allow a child with a damaged heart to decide for himself how much he can do. It was his understanding that it is impossible to assess properly the condition of a person's heart without reference to the functional reserve of the heart muscle which led him to criticise insurance companies who, on medical examination forms, ask for detailed information about the size of the heart, its sounds, its rate, its rhythm, but fail to enquire about the heart's response to exertion.

It was the lack of wisdom displayed by some practitioners in the interpretation of murmurs during the nineteenth century, that led Mackenzie to say, when speaking about the stethoscope, that it had 'not only for one hundred years hampered the progress of knowledge of heart affections, but had done more harm than good, in that many people had had the tenor of their lives altered, had been forbidden to undertake duties for which they were perfectly competent, and had been subjected to unnecessary treatment because of its "findings"'.

Since the time that Mackenzie taught his fundamental principles of cardiology to the students at the London Hospital at the beginning of this century much progress has been made and now it is widely recognised that all murmurs have to be considered on their individual merits. There is however still a tendency, amongst a minority of doctors and some parents, to play for safety with children, as may be learned from the survey of school records conducted by Bergman and Stamm, published in 1967 in the *New England Journal of Medicine*. From the records of 20,500 children in Seattle schools they found that 110 of them were supposed to have 'something wrong with the heart'. They were able to examine and study 93 of these children and found that only 18 had significant heart disease, either congenital or rheumatic, whereas the remaining 75 had 'no present evidence' of heart disease, a group which they referred to as 'cardiac non-disease'. They found that 6 of the 18 children with cardiac disease and 30 of the 75 with no cardiac disease had had their activities unnecessarily restricted: this was done in 53 per cent of the cases on medical advice and in the remainder because of parents' confusion about advice given or because they thought it was in their children's interest. A disturbing feature of the survey was that it showed that the disability from 'cardiac non-disease' was greater than from actual heart disease—a pointed reminder of the necessity for skilled assessment of heart murmurs, because, as the late Dr Charles Cameron maintained, health is an exclusion diagnosis and only those with a profound knowledge of disease are in a position to diagnose health.

10

The generation of electricity in the heart

A STUDY of the electrical changes which occur in heart muscle not only has been of great help in understanding the mechanism underlying many cardiac disorders, but has also led to the development in the early part of this century of an apparatus of the utmost importance in their diagnosis. Further, in more recent years, it has resulted in the invention of a machine capable of delivering short sharp electrical shocks to the heart muscle in certain cases of disordered rhythm.

Experiments designed to study the properties of electricity became popular from about the middle of the seventeenth century, after Otto von Guericke, the Burgomaster of Magdeburg in Prussia, invented a machine whereby appreciable amounts could be generated by friction. His apparatus consisted of a rotating globe of sulphur which became highly charged with electricity when rubbed against the hand. In 1745 Cuneus, a physicist in Leyden, electrified a jar of water by inserting into it an iron rod attached to a similar type of friction machine but when he tried to remove the rod with one hand without letting go of the jar with the other, much to his surprise he received a severe shock. Pieter van Musschenbroek, his teacher, attempted to repeat the procedure, only to be rendered unconscious. It was quickly realised that these unfortunate accidents were due to the jar having acted as a condenser or collector of electricity but at the same time the practical value of storing electricity in what was from then known as a Leyden jar was appreciated.

It was not long before scientists began to draw comparisons between naturally occurring electricity and that artificially produced by their machines. They noted the similarity between the lightning in the sky and the sparks produced by their electrical apparatus, also between the noise of thunder and the crackle of a spark. But it was the American, Benjamin Franklin, who proved that lightning and man-made electrical sparks are identical when in 1752 he succeeded at Philadelphia in charging a Leyden jar with natural electricity by attaching it to a kite which he flew among thunderclouds.

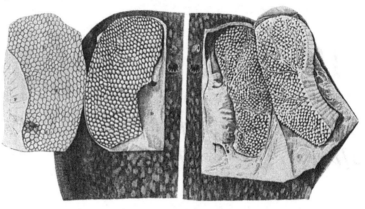

An illustration by John Hunter in the Philosophical Transactions of the Royal Society, *volume 63 (1773–4) depicting the electric organs of the torpedo fish*

Interest had already been focused on another natural source of electricity when in 1676 Bancroft suggested that the shock produced by a torpedo fish might be electrical in origin. This phenomenon had been known for centuries, the ancient Greeks having used the shock produced by this fish in the treatment of epilepsy and headaches. Accurate accounts of the skate-like torpedo fish, also of the electric eel, were given in 1773 by John Hunter and by Jan Ingenhouz, a Dutch engineer who came to London to study some of the relationships between animal and plant life with Hunter. About the same time John Walsh gave an account of the torpedo fish found around the coast of England and, because the numbing effect of their sting was similar to the shock from a Leyden jar, concluded that the fish must be capable of releasing compressed electrical fluid.

This knowledge, that the bodies of certain animals are capable of generating electricity, was undoubtedly an important factor in stimulating Galvani's interest when his attention was drawn to some unexpected reactions in an experimental animal. Luigi Galvani (1737–98) was a skilled anatomist who was first a lecturer and then professor at the University of Bologna. He is best known for his original work in electrophysiology which formed the basis for the eventual understanding of the part played by electricity in controlling the action of the heart. His private life, however, was marred by certain unfortunate events: his wife and many of his family predeceased him; he was deprived of his possessions because of an unwillingness to swear allegiance to Napoleon's Cisalpine Republic in northern Italy, and finally was afflicted by a long and painful illness from which he died at the age of sixty.

His interest in electricity began when, as a medical student, his Professor of Medicine, Leo Caldani, demonstrated that isolated nerve-muscle preparations could be stimulated by the electrical

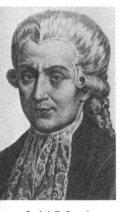

Luigi Galvani (1737–98)

discharge from a Leyden jar. But it was the chance observation of one of his own students that led him to investigate the subject of nerve-muscle contractions more closely himself. Galvani had dissected a frog and being, he admitted, preoccupied with other matters, placed it on the same table as a friction machine. Although the animal was some distance from the machine, when an assistant touched a nerve in its leg with a scalpel the muscles underwent violent contractions. Another assistant thought he had observed a similar phenomenon on some other occasion after a spark had been discharged from the machine. They therefore drew Galvani's attention to their observations whereupon he decided to repeat the experiment. In a classic monograph published in 1791 he reports that when he applied his scalpel to one of the main nerves in the frog's leg, at the same time as his assistant generated an electric spark with the machine, the muscles immediately contracted. Influenced by Franklin's observations he then attempted to repeat the experiment using electricity generated by thunderclouds. For this purpose he hung a number of frogs' legs on the balcony of his house, fastening them to the ironwork by a copper wire hooked under the femoral nerve. He noted with surprise that every time the legs touched the balcony the muscles contracted even when there was no storm in the atmosphere. At first he wondered if this was due to the escape to earth of some atmospheric electricity already accumulated in the frogs' tissues, but found he could obtain similar contractions indoors by pressing a brass hook against a leg placed on an iron plate. From this he concluded that there must be electricity stored inside the muscle which could be discharged by the apposition of two similar metals. Doubt, however, was thrown on this supposition by Alessandro Volta, Professor of Natural Philosophy at Pavia, who showed that electricity is generated when metals are placed together but was unable, with the electrical measuring apparatus available at that time, to detect any natural electricity emanating from animal tissues. He therefore concluded that the response of the muscles in Galvani's frogs was not caused by innate animal electricity but was in fact due to an electrical discharge created by a circuit between two different metals.

Although Volta was correct as to the manner in which electricity had been generated in Galvani's experiment, Galvani remained convinced that electricity does arise spontaneously within the body and therefore devised other experiments, the results of which were published in 1794. One of the most important was his 'Experiment without Metal' where he took a muscle with the nerve attached and observed that when he placed the free end of this nerve on an injured part of another muscle the first one underwent contraction. The controversy between Galvani and Volta was resolved in 1797 when

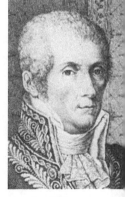

*Alessandro Volta
(1745–1827)*

the German scientist, Alexander von Humboldt, was able to confirm that Volta was right in his belief that electricity is generated by the interaction of different metals but also that Galvani was correct in his assumption that there is a biological source of electricity. As the amount of natural electricity in animal tissues is small it was some years before an instrument of sufficient sensitivity to measure it was constructed. In the meantime, Volta conducted experiments to determine the best method of producing electricity by placing different metals in contact, and found that the amount generated is substantially increased when a large number of pieces of metal are piled on top of one another. The Voltaic pile, constructed in 1799, consisting of thirty to sixty pieces of either silver or copper and an equal number of pieces of either tin or zinc, arranged in pairs and separated by paper strips soaked in salt water, gave a strong flow of electricity when the ends of the 'pile' were joined together by a wire. This was the prototype of modern batteries and the first instrument to produce an electric current.

The first man to apply the principles of electricity and magnetism formulated by Gilbert and to observe the effects of an electric current generated by a Voltaic pile on a magnet was Hans Christian Oersted, Professor of Natural Philosophy in the University of Copenhagen. He, in 1820, showed that when a pivoted magnet, or compass needle, is placed near a wire linking the two ends of a Voltaic pile, the needle is deflected so that it lies transversely to the wire; the direction of movement being dependent on whether the needle is placed above or below the wire. It was this clear demonstration of a magnetic field surrounding an electrical circuit that led André-Marie Ampère to devise an instrument capable of measuring an electric current quantitatively. The efficiency of the instrument was improved by Johannes Schweigger who caused a current to flow through a number of wires wound on to a frame inside which was placed a magnetic needle freely suspended on a vertical pivot. This was the prototype of modern galvanometers and was made still more sensitive when Leopoldo Nobili of Florence modified it in 1825 in such a way that it became possible for him at last to measure such small amounts of electricity that he could demonstrate its presence in a nerve-muscle preparation of a frog.

It was the use of such sensitive galvanometers that enabled the Italian physicist, Carlo Matteucci, in 1838, to show that generation of electricity also occurs in heart muscle. The next step in our understanding of the electrical activity in heart muscle was when Kölliker and Müller placed the nerve of a nerve-muscle preparation of a frog on the surface of a beating heart and observed that the frog's leg contracted with each beat of the heart. They were, therefore, using animal tissue as a galvanometer. The first instrument for measuring the electrical changes in heart muscle both on contraction and at rest was the rheotome invented by the German physicist Emil Du Bois-Reymond but this was mostly used in studies of the exposed hearts of animals. It was in 1875 that Gabriel Lippmann first devised the instrument capable of recording the electrical changes in the heart of an intact animal. His inspiration for the design of this instrument occurred when on a visit to Heidelberg University in 1873 he was shown a routine laboratory experiment used for teaching students. The experiment consisted of covering a drop of mercury with dilute sulphuric acid, then touching it lightly with an iron nail and watching the mercury first contract and then return to its original shape as the nail was withdrawn. The accepted teaching was that the iron in some way changed the electrical conditions existing between the mercury and the acid. Applying the principles involved in this experiment he constructed in 1875 a simple, inexpensive electrical manometer consisting of a capillary glass tube containing a column of mercury in contact with dilute sulphuric acid. With this instrument he could measure the direction and force of the electrical potential when a current was passed through it by observing the movement of the meniscus of the mercury column.

Augustus Waller used the same instrument to measure the electrical discharge from the hearts of animals without opening the chest wall and later to make similar measurements with the human heart. Waller, who was born in Paris, first studied in Geneva, then at Aberdeen and later in London, before becoming a lecturer in physiology at the London School of Medicine for Women, followed by a similar appointment at St Mary's Hospital, Paddington. In 1902 the Senate of the University of London established a physiology laboratory with Waller as the Director.

It was while he was a lecturer at St Mary's Hospital that in 1877 he gave an important demonstration of the use of the capillary electrometer in the study of electrical changes which occur in the human heart, before a group of distinguished physiologists including Willem Einthoven of Leyden. In Waller's report of this published in the *Journal of Physiology* that year, he explains that when a pair of electrodes are strapped to the front and back of the chest and connected with a Lippmann's capillary electrometer there is a slight but definite movement of the mercury with each beat of the heart due to changes in the electrical potential. The usefulness of the capillary electrometer, however, was limited as the inertia of the mercury did not enable its movements to reflect accurately the electrical changes accompanying the heart's action so that the curves produced on the photographic plate were not truly representative.

Fortunately for medical science, developments were taking place in other directions. Advances in underwater communications had been going on since 1845 when a telegraph cable was first laid under the English Channel. William Thomson, later Lord Kelvin, published in 1856 his invention of a mirror galvanometer for receiving telegraphic messages and the following year was one of the leading scientists responsible for laying the first Atlantic underwater cable. This was followed by others but instruments for receiving the telegraphic messages were not entirely satisfactory until 1897 when Ader in Paris invented what is now known as the string galvanometer.

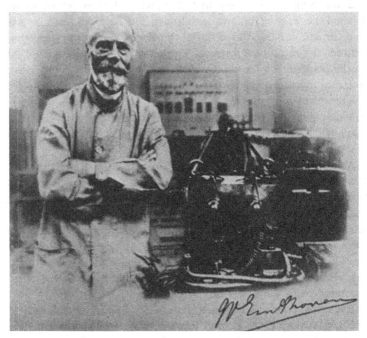

Willem Einthoven with his original string galvanometer in his laboratory at Leyden

Willem Einthoven (1860–1927), professor of physiology at Leyden University, not only had the brilliant conception that this instrument might be used to record the electrical impulses arising in the heart but also constructed an improved and more sensitive modification of the apparatus. From his description of this instrument, published in 1903, it may be seen that the essential component was a thin silver-coated quartz filament stretched like a string in a strong magnetic field. When an electric current was passed through this quartz filament the latter underwent a movement which could be observed

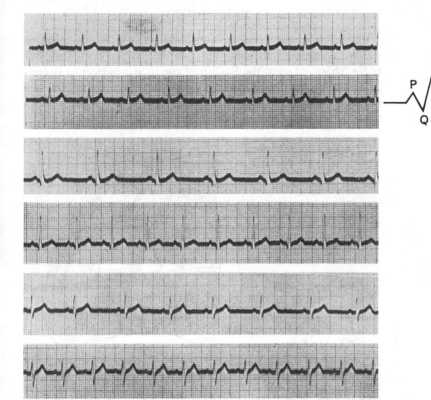

Electrocardiograms of six persons traced by means of the string galvanometer by Willem Einthoven. The diagram shows the characteristic P, Q, R, S and T waves described in the text

and photographed by means of considerable magnification. He pointed out that the string galvanometer had definite advantages over the capillary electrometer because of its greater sensitivity and it is Einthoven's galvanometer which is used to this day for recording electrocardiographs. The original instrument, was huge but now the apparatus need be no larger than a tape-recorder.

From the beginning the deflections of the filament and the speed of movement of the photographic plate were kept within arbitrary limits defined by an international committee so that workers in all parts of the world could compare their findings. Also the deflections produced with every beat of the heart were designated P, Q, R, S, and T, a nomenclature which has been continued since. The P wave is caused by contraction of the atria; the Q, R and S waves by the contraction of ventricles and the T wave by the relaxation of the ventricles. The electrocardiographs reproduced from Einthoven's original paper show the high quality of the tracings which he was able to obtain from the outset.

Einthoven was awarded the Nobel Prize in 1924 for his invention which has so greatly advanced the scientific study of cardiology, but as Sir Thomas Lewis, the English physician and pioneer in electro-cardiography, said in referring to Einthoven, 'Honours were to him a smaller recompense than was the knowledge of the benefits which his long and arduous work had conferred upon his fellow men'.

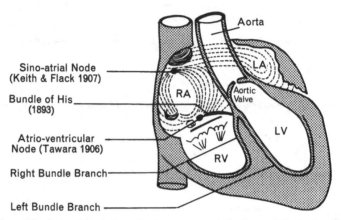

Sino-atrial Node
(Keith & Flack 1907)

Bundle of His
(1893)

Atrio-ventricular
Node (Tawara 1906)

Right Bundle Branch

Left Bundle Branch

Aorta

LA

Aortic
Valve

RA

LV

RV

Anatomy of the electrical conducting system of the heart. The broken lines represent electrical impulses which, arising in the sino-atrial node, travel out-wards through both atria and downwards to the atrio-ventricular node. From there they are transmitted via a bundle of special conduction tissues (the bundle of His) and its left and right branches to both ventricles

The smooth functioning of the heart depends on the regular production of electrical impulses which, arising from a focal point in the upper part of the right auricle, spread to the rest of the heart along specialised conduction tissue. The discovery of this tissue was the result of systematic histological work of four men. When it was discovered that the heart was supplied with nerves connected to the brain it was thought that they must control the heart's action in the same way as they control the contraction of other muscles. The first person to challenge this theory was Wilhelm His, Junior, who at the age of thirty, when working at the University of Leipzig, showed, in 1893, from embryological studies, that the heart starts beating before the nerves from the brain are developed. He thus proved that the muscle itself is capable of producing its own rhythmic stimuli but why it starts beating in the first place is as mysterious as life itself. Next he investigated the manner in which the stimuli are conducted to the various parts of the heart and found, on microscopic examina-tion, a bundle of specialised tissues connecting the auricular and ventricular septal walls. The next contribution came from Suano Tawara, a Japanese student who was working with the famous

German pathologist, Ludwig Aschoff. Tawara, in 1906, in the course of tracing out the fibres previously described by His, identified a node of special cells, known as the atrio-ventricular node, which acts as a relay station for the passage of impulses from the auricles to the ventricles. This was followed the next year by the contribution of two British scientists, Sir Arthur Keith, the distinguished anatomist and Martin Flack, a physiologist. It was they who found a little node of distinctive cells in the wall of the right atrium near the entrance

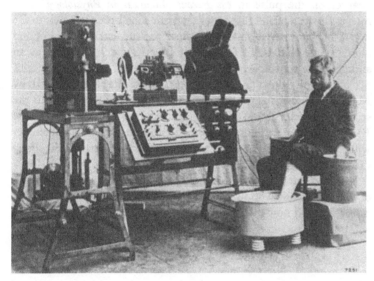

The electrocardiograph used by Sir Thomas Lewis in 1912. The instrument incorporated Einthoven's string galvanometer, and it was the first electro-cardiograph to be made by the Cambridge Instrument Company

of the superior vena cava and correctly surmised that this must be the focal point from which all the stimuli for the heart's action originate. The truth of this was confirmed and the electrical nature of these impulses demonstrated by the studies of Sir Thomas Lewis with his Einthoven's galvanometer a few years later.

Thomas Lewis (1881–1945) the son of a wealthy mining engineer in Cardiff, was first educated at Clifton College and later studied medicine at University College, Cardiff, graduating in 1904. Two years later he was appointed to the staff of the London Chest Hospital in Victoria Park, and at the same time began a private consultant practice in Queen Anne Street. The turning point in his career occurred in 1910 when he was appointed the first Beit Memorial Fellow, as this enabled him to commence the long series of important experimental laboratory investigations and clinical

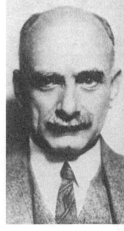

Sir Thomas Lewis (1881–1945)

research which made him famous. In 1913 he became a consulting physician to University College Hospital in London and three years later gave up private practice on his appointment as the first whole-time research physician to the staff of the Medical Research Council, with a ward and laboratories provided for him by University College Hospital.

His observations, at the age of twenty-five, on the influence of respiration on the arterial and venous pulses so impressed the physiologist Leonard Hill that he asked Lewis to contribute a chapter on the pulse in his *Recent Advances in Physiology*. This interest in the rate and rhythm of the heart soon brought Lewis to the notice of James Mackenzie, who had recently arrived in London after having established for himself a world-wide reputation as an authority on cardiac irregularities from studies he had made with his polygraph whilst in general practice in Burnley. Inspired by Mackenzie, Lewis became a member of a group who continued the study of the disorders of rhythm with the aid of electrocardiography. For this purpose he bought his own Einthoven String Galvanometer which he purchased for £120 and installed in a cellar at University College Hospital.

The fascinating story of Sir James Mackenzie's study of disorders of the pulse while working alone in general practice, its influence on cardiology and how it led to further advances by Sir Thomas Lewis will be described in the following chapter.

11

Disorders of rate and rhythm

IT is surprising that, considering the healthy heart pumps about six litres of blood every minute under considerable pressure into the circulation, its action is so smooth as usually not to be noticed. Disorders of its rate and rhythm with awareness of its action may be the result of heart disease, but also may be experienced by people with normal hearts such as when, in response to exertion, nervous stress, fever, or at times for no obvious reason, there is a sudden increase in force and rate; or when, for some innocent reason, the action becomes irregular. The symptoms are always alarming to the person concerned and for a long time such disorders were considered to be invariably of serious significance. It was only during the last century that the benign nature of some of them was appreciated. The ability to distinguish between the various types of disorder was a great advance but one that took a long time to develop.

The study of the pulse first depended on being able to measure its rate. The physicians in ancient China counted it against their own rate of breathing and Herophilus used the clepsydra, or water clock. In the seventeenth century Sandorio of Padua devised an ingenious string pendulum, the rate of whose swing could be varied by shortening the cord so that by adjusting the length of the cord the leaden weight could be made to swing in time with the pulse; the length of the cord read on a scale gave the rate of the swing and therefore the rate of the pulse. The accurate assessment of the pulse however really had to wait until Sir John Floyer, at the beginning of the eighteenth century, introduced the pulse watch which ran for a minute. His essay *The Physician's Pulse-Watch*, published in 1707, contained some remarkable observations. The influence of food, drink, tobacco, age, as well as changes in the atmosphere, are all discussed. He said, 'Custom has made tobacco part of our diet: one pipe raises the pulse five beats in a morning in one minute.' Also, he observed, 'the most natural pulse will have from seventy to seventy-five in a minute in perfect health. The lowest I have counted is fifty-five, the highest one hundred and thirty-two.' He hoped that all young physicians would, by the use of a pulse watch 'discern all those dangerous exorbitances which are caused by an irregular diet, violent passions, and a slothful life'.

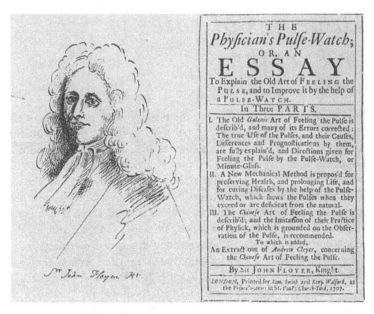

Sir John Floyer (1649–1734) and the title-page of The Physician's Pulse-Watch

It is interesting that the slowest rate which Floyer encountered was fifty-five. The resting pulse rate of athletes is often about this; undue slowing of an otherwise healthy heart may also occur in the presence of jaundice, raised intracranial pressure, or underactivity of the thyroid gland. A fall in the rate to forty or thirty beats in a minute or even less may occur but is usually then the result of disease within the heart itself. A rate as slow as this, particularly when damage to the conduction tissue prevents any increase in response to stress or exertion, often leads to an inadequate supply of blood to the brain with resultant recurring episodes of unconsciousness and convulsions. Attention was first drawn to this condition, now known as 'heart block',* by Giovanni Morgagni, the Professor of Medicine at

*Heart block: A disorder in which the ventricles beat very slowly—now known to occur when the electrical impulses from the atria are prevented from flowing into the ventricles because of disease in the electrical conduction tissue of the heart.

Padua. Morgagni contributed much to our knowledge of disease because of his practice, over many years, of conscientiously correlating the clinical appearances of disease with those he found at post-mortem examinations. As was the custom in his time he recorded

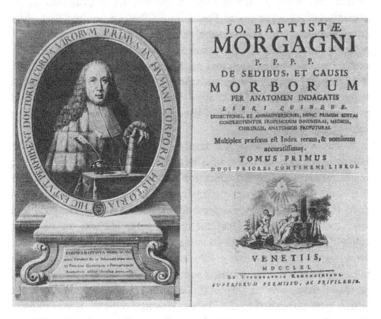

Giovanni Morgagni and the title-page of De Sedibus et Causis Morborum

his observations in letters to a friend. These letters, seventy of them in all, were then returned to Morgagni, revised, and published in a huge work of five books. This work *De Sedibus et Causis Morborum* (The Seats and Causes of Diseases) was published in 1761 when he was aged seventy-nine. It was in the ninth letter, 'Which treats of epilepsy', that he gave a clear account of what must have been a case of heart block in a priest who had a convulsion for the first time at the age of sixty-eight. When Morgagni examined him he found he had a persistent marked slowness of the pulse and that it became particularly slow just before the onset of each fit. He also drew attention to the German, Marcus Gerbezius's description in 1719 of a man with 'epilepsy' accompanied by an extremely slow pulse.

The first British physician to record the association between these two conditions was Thomas Spens who published the report of a case in 1793. He described how, about 9 o'clock on the evening of 16 May 1792, he was called to the house of a fifty-four-year-old labourer who, that afternoon, had hurt himself when suddenly and unexpectedly he fell to the ground unconscious and who, later in the

day, had three similar episodes accompanied by convulsive movements of his limbs. Spens says that having listened to this story he
was much surprised on examination to find that the man's pulse rate
was only twenty-four strokes in a minute. The man then had several
further fits with at times even more violent convulsions often
precipitated by attempts to feed himself, before he died four days
later. Post-mortem examination revealed nothing abnormal except
possibly some excess fluid around the brain. Spens thought that the
pressure on the brain from this might have had a secondary effect on
the heart and caused it to beat abnormally slowly, a not unreasonable
supposition because it is known that a raised cerebrospinal fluid
pressure does cause slowing of the pulse, but not as slow as in the
case of this man.

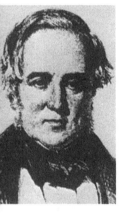

Robert Adams
(1791–1875)

It was Robert Adams, the famous Irish surgeon, in his Dublin
Hospital Reports of 1827, who was the first to appreciate that the
cerebral symptoms in this condition were due to a poor circulation to
the brain from a disorder primarily of the heart. Adams, who was
born in Dublin, became surgeon to the Jervis Street Hospital and
later to the Richmond Hospital in that city. He was an excellent
teacher whose lectures proved extremely popular with his students.
In addition he wrote many outstanding papers on diseases of the
joints and contributed, perhaps somewhat surprisingly for a surgeon
in those days, several important articles on diseases of the heart
which were published in the Dublin Hospital reports. It was in May
1819, when surgeon to the Jervis Street Hospital, that Adams
observed what is now known as heart block in a sixty-eight-year-
old Revenue officer. Adams, who saw the patient at the request of his
general practitioner following an attack of apoplexy says, 'what most
attracted my attention was the irregularity of his breathing and
remarkable slowness of the pulse, which generally ranged at the rate
of thirty in a minute'. The patient's practitioner told him that during
the past seven years the man had had at least twenty similar apoplec-
tic attacks, with each time an initial period of lethargy, confusion and
loss of memory, followed by sudden loss of consciousness often
resulting in injury. Also, that during the attacks, he had noted his
patient's pulse to be slower than usual. Adams was astute enough to
recognise that the apoplexy 'must be considered less a disease in
itself than symptomatic of one, the organic seat of which was in the
heart'. When the patient finally came to post-mortem examination
the heart muscle was found to be of poor quality and to a large extent
replaced by fat. Adams concluded that it was because the heart beat
so slowly that the brain was starved of sufficient blood hence the
lethargy, loss of memory and other cerebral symptoms. He had no
idea however what caused this slow action of the heart.

His contemporary, the physician William Stokes, however, gained a certain amount of insight into the nature of the underlying cause in such cases from an inspection of the jugular pulse and by auscultation of the heart with a stethoscope. William Stokes (1804–78) had the good fortune to have a gifted father who was, in his time, a professor of medicine in Dublin and who, in addition to his knowledge of medicine, had wide interests in the natural sciences and arts. It was a devoted family and William in particular shared many of his father's interests and accompanied him on frequent archaeological and scientific excursions. It was from this study of plant and animal life with his father that he developed powers of observation which he applied to such good effect later in his life when he turned to the investigation of disease in man. He began his medical studies in Dublin but after a short time went to Glasgow where he read chemistry for two years and then completed his medical studies in Edinburgh. It was there that he had the good fortune to come under the influence of Professor William Allison who, by his example, not only inspired his gifted pupil to become skilled in the science of medicine but also developed in him feelings of concern and compassion for his individual patients. The teaching of medicine at that time was undergoing a radical change since the introduction of the stethoscope. Stokes, while still a student, made a special study of auscultation and before he qualified as a doctor wrote an important treatise on the use of the stethoscope in the examination of the lungs. This was printed in Edinburgh in 1825, the year that he qualified, at the age of twenty-one. After this he returned to Dublin where one year later he was appointed a physician to the Meath Hospital on the retirement of his father. There is no doubt that the reputation he had established by the publication of his work on the stethoscope was greatly in his favour.

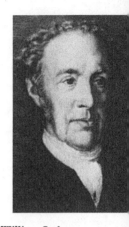

William Stokes
(1804–78)

Stokes, together with his colleague, Robert Graves, reorganised the medical teaching in Dublin so that it became internationally famous. Not only did they give outstanding formal lectures but also emphasised the importance of informal bedside teaching, not hitherto generally practised in medical schools, which enabled students to study the effects of disease at first hand. Stokes's influence on the education of medical students was enormous, insisting as he did that it was important for them to have a high standard of general education in order to avoid becoming nothing but technicians and also stressed the importance of every student receiving instruction both in surgery and in medicine rather than in one or the other as was the practise.

His first important major work, published in 1837, was a treatise on the diagnosis and treatment of diseases of the chest. This book contains numerous original observations and is profusely illustrated by pen pictures, but perhaps most important of all it brought to the attention of many English-speaking doctors for the first time the value of the stethoscope in the diagnosis of diseases of the lung. After the publication of this work he received many honours, the University of Dublin conferred on him a doctorate of medicine; the King's and Queen's College of Physicians in Ireland elected him a Fellow; the Imperial Academy of Medicine of Vienna made him an honorary member as did the Royal Medical Societies of Berlin, Leipzig, Ghent and Edinburgh. In America he was elected a member of the National Institute of Philadelphia. This enthusiastic reception of his work greatly encouraged him both as a teacher and writer and during the next ten years he directed his attention more especially to a study of the disorders of the heart. This work culminated in the publication, in 1854, of his book *The Disease of the Heart and Aorta*, a work based on the large series of original papers contributed by him in the intervening years to the *Dublin Quarterly Journal of Medical Science*.

By then, the medical profession's acceptance of Auenbrugger's method of percussion and Laënnec's auscultation, and their routine use in the examination of a patient, had unfortunately led to too much importance being attached to physical signs so that the symptoms were often ignored, or not properly evaluated. Stokes emphasised once again the importance of conscientious history-taking and pointed out that in many diseases, including those of the heart, physical signs may at times be few, when symptoms are an important indication of serious disease. Conversely, obvious signs such as loud murmurs heard with the stethoscope, in the absence of symptoms, may not be of much significance. By his insistence on the correlation of signs and symptoms he did much to promote the science of auscultation and taught how to distinguish significant cardiac murmurs; at the same time, he emphasised that listening to the patient's story was often as, or even more, important than listening to his heart. His belief that the function of the heart could best be assessed not by auscultation but by observing the response of the patient to exercise was not readily understood by the profession and its acceptance had to wait for another fifty years until emphasised by Sir James Mackenzie.

His book, famous for its accurate descriptions of pericarditis, valvular diseases and the effects on the heart of typhus fever, contains in addition his 'Observations on some cases of Permanently Slow Pulse' which had already appeared in the *Dublin Quarterly Journal of Medical Science* in 1846. This account refers to seven cases, three of which were his own, two of Robert Adams's and two under the care of other physicians. He noticed that in five of the cases there was a murmur, proved at post-mortem examination to be due to degenerative changes in the aortic valve but he argued that this could not be the cause of the abnormally slow pulse as from the other two cases he knew this could occur in its absence. Although he therefore did not know the cause, he was enabled, by shrewd clinical observations, to deduce that there is a complete dissociation of the action of the auricles and ventricles in this condition.

Blood from the upper part of the body returns to the heart by flowing through the jugular veins in the neck to the right auricle, and careful inspection of the pulsation in these veins will give information about the action of the auricles. Although the application of this to clinical medicine was not widely employed until Mackenzie developed the method towards the end of the century, Stokes appreciated its value and must have been one of the first men to make such observations even if he did not always understand their significance. Thus in his account of his first case he writes:

Within the present month [June] this patient has been again admitted into hospital. The cardiac phenomena remain as before but a new symptom has appeared, namely a very remarkable pulsation in the right jugular vein. This is most evident when the patient is lying down. The number of the reflex pulsations is difficult to be established, but they are more than double the number of the manifest ventricular contractions.

It was this observation, and the hearing of muffled sounds in addition to slow distinct ones on listening with a stethoscope, that led him to realise that in this condition the auricles and ventricles are out of phase and that the ventricles beat regularly in their own slow time completely dissociated from the faster beating of the auricles. This was later confirmed by Mackenzie with the help of his polygraph and shown by Thomas Lewis from electrocardiographic studies at the beginning of this century to be due to a block in the conduction tissue preventing electrical impulses arising in the right auricle from reaching the ventricles.

Much work has been done since Stokes's time to discover the cause of the block. Some cases are due to congenital errors of development, some the result of damage from coronary thrombosis, and in recent years some from damage incurred during heart surgery. But, in about half the cases, a peculiar type of scarring, the cause of which is unknown, is found invading the conduction tissue while the heart muscle and coronary arteries remain healthy. The incidence of chronic complete heart block is difficult to assess but Siddons and Sowton in 1967 estimated that fifty cases per million population arise each year so that in the United Kingdom there would be about 2,500 new cases per year.

Treatment of the symptoms of this condition, sometimes eponymously known as Stokes-Adams attacks, has for long consisted of stimulating the action of the ventricles by sympathomimetic

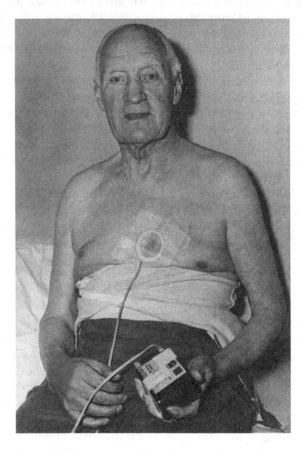

Patient whose heart rate was abnormally slow because of a block in the electrical conduction tissue (complete heart block) fitted with an artificial pacemaker. A ring-shaped coil with leads connected to the heart has been implanted inside the chest. A stimulating pulse is induced in the coil taped to the patient's chest immediately over it. This external coil is connected to a battery-powered pulse generator carried in a pocket or on a belt

drugs* such as isoprenaline or ephedrine. On occasions these fail to control the symptoms and for such cases there has been a dramatic

*Sympathomimetic drugs—drugs which mimic the effects of stimulation of the sympathetic part of the autonomic nervous system.

advance in recent years with the invention of apparatus capable of inducing artificial electrical stimuli in the muscle of the ventricle. Such an instrument, known as an artificial pacemaker, is usually connected to the heart by an insulated wire passed through the jugular vein with its platinum tip impacted in the apex of the right ventricle. The insertion of the wire needs much skill and the patient has to have the apparatus regularly checked in a well-equipped cardiac laboratory once every three months. More recently an external pacemaker has been developed, illustrated opposite.

The distressing symptoms associated with an abnormally fast pulse known as palpitations (from the Latin *palpitare*—frequent) was discussed at length by James Hope in his textbook on heart disease published in 1831. He said that there were few affections which excited more alarm and anxiety in the minds of patients than this, and castigated his medical colleagues for taking the view that it is impossible to tell in any particular person whether palpitations are or are not of any significance. He considered that the problem could readily be resolved by the exclusion of serious underlying organic disease from a proper history and the skilful use of percussion and auscultation. He pointed out that amongst people with healthy hearts, palpitations are common in nervy individuals and are often brought on by dyspepsia, anxiety, overwork and what he called venereal excesses. He made the important observation that palpitations of a benign character always become less evident on exertion, and warned practitioners that although palpitations are often associated with indigestion it is necessary to remember that dyspepsia itself may be a symptom of heart disease. Although Hope's teaching was extremely wise, it was not until James Mackenzie applied himself to the problem later in the century that disorders of the rhythm of the heart became properly understood.

First, however, reference must be made to the work of Pierre Carl Édouard Potain, who made a special study of the pulsation in the neck veins and who, from records of these traced on smoked paper, was able to show that the movements transmitted to the veins by the auricles could be distinguished from others transmitted by the ventricles. Potain was a gifted investigator who, when he was an associate professor of the Faculty of Medicine of Paris, read a paper to the Medical Society of the Paris Hospitals at a meeting on 24 May 1867, 'On the movements and sounds that take place in the jugular veins'. Firstly, he described what he had learned from many years of visual inspection of the jugular veins and then showed how he had learned to record these pulsations on paper. He acknowledged work already done on the subject by Bamberger, Geigel and Friedreich in Germany, who had made similar recordings using the pulse

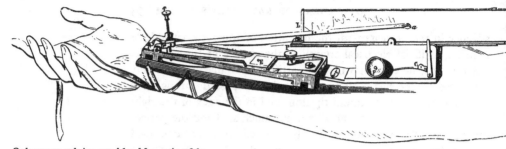

Sphygmograph invented by Marey in 1863

writer or sphygmograph* invented by his French colleague Étienne Jules Marey in 1863. This instrument had been devised for recording the amplitude and duration of the radial pulse and the German workers found technical difficulties when they attempted to use it on neck veins. Potain therefore modified the instrument; he placed a small glass funnel on the neck to act as a stethoscope, and by connecting it to a length of rubber tubing was able to transmit the impulses from the vein to a drum which was attached to a lever so that the pulsations could be recorded on the smoked paper of the sphygmograph. At the same time this instrument was attached in the usual way to the radial artery. By this method he was able to get a simultaneous tracing of the jugular pulse and the radial pulse. Not content with this he next placed another funnel on the chest so that he could now record the impulses of the heart alongside the other two. From these tracings he was able to show how the pulsations in the neck veins reflect the movement of the chambers of the heart. He demonstrated two sharp elevations in the jugular pulse; one due to contraction of the right auricle followed immediately by another due to contraction of the left ventricle. These observations were of fundamental importance but Potain did not proceed from there to apply this knowledge in analysing the various disorders of rate and rhythm as James Mackenzie did some years later in England.

James Mackenzie (1853–1925), one of the most outstanding physicians at the turn of the century, was born on a farm in Scone, Scotland. He was a pupil first at the village school and later at Perth Grammar School, which he left earlier than planned because he found routine learning difficult. At the age of fifteen he became an apprentice in a local chemist's shop. It was there that his contact with the neighbouring general practitioners convinced him that he wished to become a doctor himself and at twenty-one went to Edinburgh to study medicine. Working for examinations did not come easily to him for, as he said, his power of memory was not as

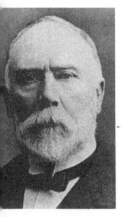

Sir James Mackenzie
(1853–1925)

*Sphygmo, from the Greek *sphugmos*—throb. Sphygmograph—instrument for recording character of pulse in a series of curves.

good as his power to reason. Nevertheless, he graduated after the completion of four years' study and a year later entered general practice as an assistant to Drs William Briggs and John Brown in Burnley, Lancashire. It was not long before he was made a partner and he stayed in the town of Burnley for the next thirty years.

Early in his career he decided to make a special study of disorders of the heart after attending a young woman who unexpectedly collapsed and died from heart failure whilst in labour. Mackenzie felt very upset as he considered this death might have been prevented if only he had recognised some sign or symptom of heart disease earlier in the pregnancy. He therefore started to examine routinely the hearts of all his women patients before, during and after pregnancy, and to his surprise found a large number of unsuspected cardiac murmurs and variations in rate and rhythm. It was accepted teaching at that time that any irregularity of the pulse was always dangerous but when he followed the progress of patients who showed evidence of dysrhythmia through their pregnancies he found that although a few developed heart failure the majority went through labour without any difficulty. He considered this could only be explained by there being several different types of irregularity, some dangerous but others harmless. In order to assist him in differentiating between them he recorded the pulses of a large number of pregnant women with the sphygmograph devised by Dudgeon. This instrument, like the one invented by Marey, when strapped to the

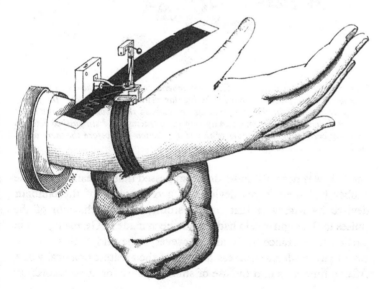

Dudgeon's sphygmograph

wrist records the movements of the radial pulse on a moving plate. He found many different types of pulse with varying rates, rhythms and wave patterns. He experienced much difficulty in interpreting these until, like Potain, though unaware of his work, he turned to a study of the jugular veins in the neck. The pulsation in these vessels is extremely difficult to observe with the naked eye and it is interesting that the steps taken by these two men to make this task easier, although completely independent, were remarkably similar. Mackenzie gummed straws on to the neck in order to magnify the movements of the veins whereas Potain in a similar fashion had used strips of coloured paper. Mackenzie then developed an instrument like that of Potain so that he could record these pulsations on the smoked paper of a sphygmograph. Finally, he too devised a polygraph so that recordings with three pens gave simultaneous tracings of the jugular pulse, radial pulse and pulsations of the heart in the

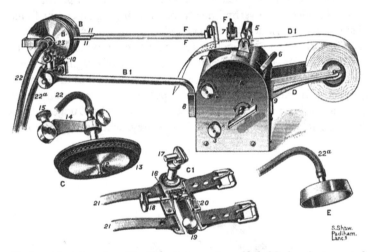

Mackenzie's ink polygraph. This instrument enabled Mackenzie to record tracings of pulse waves arising in the jugular veins in the neck and the radial artery at the wrist at the same time as he recorded the movements of the heart against the chest wall. From an analysis of these tracings he distinguished between many different types of disorder of the heart's action long before the more direct method of electrocardiography was invented

chest. It was not until some time had passed that he learned that the rubber ball used in his device was a reinvention of the tambour devised by Marey or that similar studies of the behaviour of the pulses in the jugular vein had already been made in Germany, and in particular in France by Potain. However, as he said, their work was essentially academic whereas his was of the greatest practical value. After a time he found the use of smoked paper for these recordings unsatisfactory and with the help of Mr Shaw, a watchmaker in the village of Padiham near Bolton, he constructed a polygraph whose tracings were recorded on paper in ink; an apparatus known to this day as Mackenzie's ink polygraph. With this apparatus he distinguished three waves in his tracings of the jugular vein and by comparing the timing of these with the arterial pulse wave came to the same conclusion as Potain, that the first two arise from contraction of the right auricle and the left ventricle respectively, but the third, now known to be due to a rise in pressure in the vein when the right auricle fills with blood prior to its contraction, remained for a time obscure to him.

He decided to use the polygraph in order to study the action of the right auricle and the left ventricle in cases with irregularity of the heart beat. The first patient he investigated in this manner was a man complaining of having 'missed' beats. Mackenzie, from a simultaneous tracing of the jugular and radial pulses, was immediately able to see that whereas the right auricle was beating regularly the left ventricle was from time to time contracting earlier than it should. These extra beats, or extrasystoles as they were called by Mackenzie, because they come too soon in the cardiac cycle are weaker than normal beats and for this reason are not transmitted to the radial pulse so that the patient gets the feeling that a beat has been missed. Other patients complained of an intermittent thumping in the chest due to the excessive force with which the ventricles contract following an extrasystole. This is because more blood than usual has time to enter the ventricles during the abnormally long pause between an extrasystole and the next normal beat. Today every doctor is so familiar with extrasystoles as to make them commonplace, but for Mackenzie it was a wonderful experience to be able to demonstrate for the first time, with the help of his apparatus, the mechanism of the irregularity.

I can remember [wrote Mackenzie thirty years later] the excitement which filled me when I fully appreciated this discovery. When, however, I announced my discovery, no one believed it and no one accepted it even although I sent my papers describing this and other observations to the leading physiologists of the day ... notwithstanding the complete indifference with which my work was viewed, I knew that I was getting at the truth.

This was the turning point in Mackenzie's career. Up to then he had been diffident and underrated his abilities but now at last he realised his worth. He saw clearly that his future life's work must be to make an accurate analysis of all the signs and symptoms of heart disease, and then to assess their relative significance by a methodical long-term follow-up of the patients affected. First, he began by following up all the patients in whom he had demonstrated the presence of extrasystoles and found that after six years those who had only this disorder without any other evidence of heart disease were alive and well, many of them having performed heavy manual labour and a number of women having had uneventful pregnancies. At a meeting in London, where he addressed a group of heart specialists, he was able to say with conviction, 'I have never known any harm befall anyone in whom this irregularity was the only sign of departure from the normal'. Immediately, a specialist rose and said, 'I had four patients whose pulses were irregular in the way described by Dr Mackenzie. They all died.' To which Mackenzie retorted, 'I had four hundred patients with bald heads. They all died. But it was not the baldness of their heads that killed them.' Time has shown that as Mackenzie taught, extrasystoles occurring alone are innocent and extremely common. Their incidence increases with age, they may occur only occasionally or as frequently as every other beat, they are particularly noticeable at night when the patient is lying in bed and as Hope pointed out at the beginning of the last century, they disappear with exercise. Often, on the other hand, they come on after exertion or are triggered off by tiredness, emotional stress, fever, or over indulgence in alcohol, tea or tobacco. They may, on the other hand, accompany heart disease and in such cases the prognosis depends on the seriousness of the underlying cardiac disorder. They not infrequently occur when the heart muscle is deprived of oxygen due to narrowing of the coronary arteries and their appearance following a coronary thrombosis often heralds the particularly dangerous disturbance of rhythm known as ventricular tachycardia.* Their occurrence in patients under treatment with digitalis indicates that the heart muscle is being poisoned by an overdose of the drug and is an indication therefore for it to be temporarily discontinued. Mackenzie's recognition that extrasystoles in the absence of serious heart disease are in themselves of no importance, was a great advance as it has enabled many patients to be confidently reassured and spared the unnecessary imposition of restricted activity.

Children too benefited from his work; it is not uncommon for a child's pulse to increase in rate during inspiration, and to slow again during expiration. This type of irregularity, up to then considered to be of serious import, engaged Mackenzie's attention once he had resolved the problem of extrasystoles. He reviewed the patients whose pulse recordings five or six years earlier had shown an increased rate on inspiration and found that all of them, without exception, had remained fit. He found that most were children, in contrast to his patients with extrasystoles who were predominantly

*Tachy from the Greek *takhus* – swift.

adult. Thus he called the irregularity of pulse affected by breathing, 'the youthful type' to distinguish it from the various forms of extra-systole which he referred to as 'the adult type' of irregularity.

I found [he wrote] the youthful type most distinct in perfectly healthy children and youths ... I watched those who showed this irregularity grow into manhood and womanhood and observed many of them during tem-porary illness and during periods of severe bodily effort. They never showed any signs of cardiac weakness, even when they were engaged in hard manual labour. I therefore concluded that the condition was a physiological one.

The medical profession however was slow to accept Mackenzie's teaching so that some years later, after he had relinquished general practice in Burnley to become a London Harley Street specialist, one of the first patients brought to him was a girl who had been kept in bed for three months because of an irregular pulse. Finding it was no more than the benign youthful type of irregularity he had the difficult task of persuading the parents to allow her to lead a normal life. Another patient he saw about the same time, a boy, had not only been made to stay in bed for several months but had then been for-bidden to play all games; following this he had been taken to a fashionable continental clinic where for many months he languished and was then given a prolonged course of injections by another specialist before his parents, having been told he was incurable, brought him home. As a last desperate hope they consulted Mackenzie who once again, finding the irregularity to be no more than the youthful type, at once recommended that the boy should be allowed to live normally. This he did, and Mackenzie had the satis-faction of following his progress during an active school life and as a soldier in the First World War.

Advice such as Mackenzie gave to these parents sounds easy, but it was revolutionary in his day and was the result of fifteen to twenty years' observation of very large numbers of patients after having first obtained and analysed the recordings of their pulses. The medical profession was impressed by the cleverness of his recording apparatus but was far slower to appreciate that the information he gained from it was of little value without long periods of diligent follow-up. On one occaion he regretfully commented that if he had discovered some remedy which cured the condition he would have received wide-spread praise but because he had only shown that the irregularity was of no importance, the value of his advance was not appreciated.

There was yet a third type of disturbance of rhythm which had puzzled Mackenzie for a long time in which the pulse was so irregular that every beat was of a different strength and every pause between each beat of a different length. He had kept tracings taken from a number of these patients over the years together with a careful account of their progress. He found that after six years many were dead, others were in obvious heart failure and only a few in comparative good health. There could be no doubt that this disorder was entirely different from the other two and of a dangerous type. When Mackenzie studied the tracings of the jugular pulse in this group of patients he found that the first of the three usual waves was missing, that is to say there was no evidence of auricular contraction. This was very puzzling and on consulting his records he found that 80 per cent of his patients who suffered from this particular type of disturbance of the pulse had suffered in the past from acute rheumatic fever. He decided, therefore, that next time he had a patient with this disease he would follow the progress of the case from the early acute stage to see whether any spectacular change took place when this irregularity of pulse appeared which might throw light on its causation. His opportunity arose when a woman he had first seen in an acute attack of rheumatic fever in 1880 and who had had recurrences in 1883 and 1884 consulted him again in 1890. On that occasion he found that the pulse was regular in rhythm but on auscultation he heard a murmur just before the first of the two normal heart sounds, that is, a presystolic murmur, which he correctly interpreted as arising from progressive scarring and narrowing of the mitral valve between the left auricle and the left ventricle. This patient with mitral stenosis was now kept under careful observation and regularly examined until 1898 when her condition suddenly deteriorated, heart failure appeared and when Mackenzie examined her he found she had developed complete irregularity of her pulse; also for the first time he noticed that the presystolic murmur had vanished and the first of the three waves in her jugular pulse had disappeared. He knew that the presystolic murmur was produced by the contraction of the left auricle forcing blood through a narrowed valve into the left ventricle and that the first wave of the jugular pulse was caused by contraction of the right auricle. As both had now disappeared he concluded that neither auricle was contracting; a belief that seemed to receive support when a year later his patient died and at post-mortem examination her auricles were found to be so greatly distended and thin-walled as to be quite incapable of exercising any pressure on their content. He therefore referred to this dangerous type of irregularity in 1902 as paralysis of the auricles. Doubt as to whether this was the correct interpretation arose when at other post-mortem examinations of patients who had had this type of irregularity he found auricles with thick walls quite obviously capable of strong contractions. He therefore offered the alternative suggestion that possibly the auricles and ventricles contract synchronously in this condition with the primary stimulus for contraction arising in the auriculo-ventricular node rather than at the usual side in the wall of the right auricle. It was for this reason that for a time he erroneously referred to it as nodal rhythm. This explanation still did not satisfy him and he endeavoured to interest others who might be able to investigate the matter by experimental methods to find out exactly how the auricles do behave in this condition. It was Arthur Cushney, Professor of Pharmacology in Edinburgh, who, on a visit to Mackenzie at Burnley in 1906 first suggested to him that it might be that the auricles undergo fibrillation, a peculiar writhing movement of the muscle which he had experimentally produced in dogs. This seemed a very likely explanation especially as Thomas Lewis, not long after, found that the appearance of electrocardiographs taken from patients with this type of irregularity, were exactly comparable to electrocardiographs taken from dogs with artificially induced auricular fibrillation. Such tracings, because of the disordered rhythm of the ventricles, showed that the size and timing of the Q, R, S waves were completely irregular and in addition showed an entire absence of P waves, thus confirming that the auricles were not contracting normally. Lewis then decided to observe the peculiar movements of the auricles at first hand by examining the exposed hearts of horses with this condition. For this purpose he contacted Professor Woodruff at the Royal Veterinary College and General Smith of the Royal Army Veterinary Corps. Woodruff agreed to have a careful search made for horses with an irregular action of the heart amongst those attending the Out-Patients' Department of the Royal Veterinary College, whilst General Smith gave similar instructions to the various depots under his command. The result of this was that Lewis had five horses submitted to him with irregular hearts. His description of the result of his examination of the fifth horse which he conducted at Bulford Plain on 25 June 1910 is most instructive. It was a sixteen-year-old gelding provided by General Smith and Colonel Blenkinsop of Salisbury. Lewis confirmed the irregularity of the heart and noted that the animal became quickly short of breath after cantering a few times round a small paddock. The horse was therefore chloroformed and the heart exposed. Lewis says:

an excellent view of the beating heart was obtained, the ventricular movements were forcible and the spacing of the beats corresponded with what had been heard at the previous examination. For the horse they were rapid and irregular in the extreme ... at first no intrinsic movement could be seen in the auricle, it seemed to lie still apart from tugging transmitted from the ventricles ... closer inspection of the musculature revealed the presence of fibrillary movements ... the activity of the tissues generally was well displayed and was demonstrated to and recognised by the bystanders, including Colonel Blenkinsop.

Lewis on another occasion described the appearance of the auricles when fibrillating as being alive with movement, with rapid, minute and constant twitchings or undulatory movements observed in a multitude of small areas upon its surface.

Mackenzie, in his textbook, has an important chapter on auricular fibrillation. He describes the steps that led him to recognise this type of irregularity, the nature of the irregularity and the assistance which he had obtained from Lewis's experiments on animals and electro-cardiographic studies. He points out that in his experience there are two classes of patient very liable to develop this irregularity; firstly, those suffering from rheumatic fever, when this is complicated by the development of mitral stenosis; and secondly, elderly people with degenerative changes in their heart muscles caused by impairment of the blood supply through narrowed coronary arteries. He doesn't mention the third, now well accepted, cause of auricular fibrillation, that of overactivity of the thyroid gland. This omission is interesting because the irregularity in frequency and strength of the pulse in association with this condition had in fact been noted, although not of course recognised as fibrillation, by the Bath physician Caleb Parry at the end of the eighteenth century. Parry, in his paper on the subject entitled *Enlargement of the Thyroid Gland in Connection with Enlargement or Palpitation of the Heart* published in 1825, three years after his death, gave a description of six patients with over-activity of the thyroid gland, several of whom had fast irregular pulses; no doubt in some cases from extrasystoles superimposed on a fast regular pulse, but others, from the description, must have been fibrillating.

The final part of Mackenzie's chapter on auricular fibrillation deals with the treatment of the disorder where he points out the beneficial effect of digitalis. He says, 'it is in the treatment of auricular fibrillation that we find the great value of this drug, and I cannot speak too highly of its therapeutic action'. He administered the drug by giving sufficient of it to cause the patient to have side effects and then he reduced the dose. He says:

the best and most assured way, in cases of marked failure, is steadily to push the drug ... until a reaction is observed. Usually the digestive system is the first to crack, loss of appetite, nausea, vomiting or diarrhoea being set up, the patient usually feeling ill and miserable. If the digitalis is effective on the heart, as a rule a marked slowing of the pulse is found at the same time, or even before any digestive disturbances arise.

It was in this way that he calculated the dose for each individual which would be effective in keeping the pulse rate about eighty a minute without at the same time causing any untoward symptoms. He warned against the dangers of digitalis overdosage just as William

Withering had in the first place but the medical profession was still slow to heed the advice. Mackenzie quotes cases where heart failure had been brought under control by digitalis but too large a dosage led to sudden death and even today many cases of vomiting are due to digitalis overdosage, particularly in old people, who are peculiarly intolerant of this drug.

It is important to stress that all this valuable pioneer research work was done by Mackenzie whilst working in isolation, far removed from daily contact with heart specialists, in a busy general practice in Burnley. Although he published the results of his work in medical literature he found difficulty in being accepted among the peers of the profession at that time. He said later that, 'Sir William Osler came to see me when none other of the big physicians would have dreamed of associating with me'. While however he was ignored in his own country his fame spread to Germany, America and else-where. At an international conference of physicians held in a south-coast town four physicians from Germany enquired for Mackenzie but no one there knew that such a person existed. The Germans insisted that this was nonsense as they had already read his papers and made it clear that they had specially come to the conference to meet him. They therefore left immediately in search of Mackenzie in Burnley. His fame in Germany was such that in 1906, when Dr Arthur Hurst (later Sir Arthur Hurst) who was at that time the Radcliffe Travelling Fellow in Germany from Guy's Hospital Medical School, wrote home saying:

of all English physicians the best known and most frequently quoted in Germany is probably Dr Mackenzie of Burnley, a prophet who has hardly met, in his own country, with the recognition he deserves. The methods of studying disorders of the circulation introduced by him are much employed, and many important investigations confirming and extending his results have been published in Germany.

It was not long before Mackenzie was invited to Canada and America, as well as to many places on the Continent and soon many foreign physicians journeyed to Burnley to see his methods and discuss with him his views on cardiology. Still however he made little impact on leaders of medicine in this country. He knew that this was because he was in general practice and that nothing would change until he set up as a specialist. He was by this time fifty-four and his friends tried to advise him not to leave Burnley where he was happy, safe and content but Mackenzie knew that he had much to offer and that it was important for people to listen and he would only be able to gain an effective hearing from the vantage point of Harley Street. It was therefore with considerable courage, but with much justly earned confidence in himself, that in 1907 he uprooted his family and left his friends to come to London where he was a stranger and felt very much alone. Lady Mackenzie, at a later time, revealed that when they first moved into their new home in Bentinck Street they really were extremely poor: he had no private fortune upon which to rely whilst attempting to build up a consultant practice. He busied himself, however, writing his book on diseases of the heart which was published in 1908. This was recognised immediately as a work of great distinction and a second edition soon followed. Mackenzie has revealed that in the first year of practice in London he only earned £114 but in the second year, due to the warm reception of his book, he earned more than £1,000. More important than this, from Mackenzie's point of view, other specialists were now taking a close interest in him. Sir James Purves Stewart invited him to become a physician at the West London Hospital and Dr Frederick Price asked him to join the staff of Mount Vernon Hospital at Hampstead and also invited him to take a consulting-room in his Harley Street house. Mackenzie accepted these invitations and with his family moved out of London to Northwood in Middlesex.

Not long after this he was appointed head of a new Cardiology Department at the London Hospital and was made a Member of the Royal College of Physicians and a Fellow of the Royal Society. In addition a knighthood soon followed. These honours were conferred upon him in recognition of the advances he had made, particularly with the polygraph, in placing cardiology on a scientific basis. Mackenzie however considered this was quite wrong as he was certain that instruments such as the polygraph were a means of understanding clinical signs and not an end in themselves. It was not long after this that he received a visit in Harley Street from Professor Waller who tried to get him interested in the newly developed electrocardiograph. He recognised its possibilities but left investigation of its use to younger men. Before long important research work was being done in his department at the London Hospital, but he himself had a deep longing to get back to general practice, for although he was one of the busiest consultants in London, with a waiting-room overflowing with patients, he felt that the best place to study illness was from its earliest onset amongst people in a community rather than in the rarefied atmosphere of a laboratory or hospital wards filled with patients with advanced disease. His return to general practice was postponed by the First World War but in 1918, having reached the age of sixty-five, he abandoned his consulting practice worth at that time about £8,000 a year, in order to establish an Institute of Clinical Research amongst general practitioners. He chose St Andrews as his centre and at the first general meeting of the general practitioners there who were incorporated on to the staff of the Institute, it was resolved that the main objects of research would be the early stages of disease and that the work would primarily consist of detailed observation of symptoms and the keeping of careful records. Prolonged observation of cases would be carried out in order to discover the significance of early symptoms and research would be undertaken with a view to ascertaining the mechanism of their production. He lived to see the Institute firmly established but increasing attacks of angina limited his activities and he died on the 26 January 1925.

12

The lifeline threatened

THE health of the heart is dependent on an adequate flow of blood through the coronary arteries. These long slender vessels which arise from the root of the aorta to supply the muscle of the heart with blood, are liable to become narrowed by degenerative changes in their walls. When this occurs the blood flow to the heart muscle may only be sufficient for its needs when the body is at rest but not when the work of the heart is increased in response to stress such as exercise or emotion. In such circumstances the person affected develops angina which is a transitory but alarming constricting sensation usually across the front of the chest brought on by exertion and relieved by rest. Much worse than this is when the blood, flowing slowly through these narrowed vessels, suddenly clots. This event, known as a coronary thrombosis, is an immediate threat to the patient's life and because of the resultant serious and often extensive damage to the muscle there is prolonged agonising pain also usually across the front of the chest, which may come on at any time and is not relieved by rest. These two conditions have recently become the subject of much discussion but they are certainly not new diseases for the characteristic narrowing of the coronary arteries has been found in the mummified hearts of ancient Egyptians.

The coronary arteries received little or no attention until the publication of the *Six Tables* in 1538, an anatomical work which contained a detailed description of these vessels by Vesalius and drawings by Van Kalkar. Also there was no mention of their function until William Harvey, in *De motu cordis*, stated that this was to nourish the heart muscle. Recognition of the effect of disease in these arteries had to wait until physicians learned the great value of correlating appearances found on postmortem examination with symptoms and signs present in life. The first man to make extensive use of this method of learning was Giovanni Morgagni: in his sixteenth letter published in *De Sedibus* in 1761 he says, 'those who have dissected or inspected many [bodies] have at least learned to doubt; when others, who are ignorant of anatomy and do not take the trouble to attend to it, are in no doubt at all'. Several of the letters in *De Sedibus* relate to his studies of heart disease and in the twenty-fourth letter he describes how he found, in the body of an old man who had died from the effects of a strangulated hernia, the walls of the coronary arteries, as well as parts of several other arteries in the body so hard and thickened that it felt as if they had been replaced by bone. These changes were of such a novel character that he reports he demonstrated them to a very crowded circle of students and considered them worthy of special description in a letter. There is no mention, however, that these narrowed vessels had been the cause of any symptoms in life. He does however in addition report the post-mortem examination of a forty-two-year-old woman who suddenly died while on a tour of the Continent. She had been suffering for a long time from severe attacks of constricting chest pain with a numbness of the left arm and difficulty in breathing, precipitated by exertion and relieved by rest. Although this was a clear description of the effects of coronary artery disease the condition was not widely recognised until after William Heberden's lecture on angina pectoris to the Royal College of Physicians in 1768.

Heberden, unlike most of his colleagues in the eighteenth century, who spent their time arguing about the theories of ancient writers, studied disease at the bedside and, like Sydenham in the previous century, was enabled by detailed observation of his patients to make many original contributions to our knowledge of disease. Born in London he received his early education at the Grammar School of St Saviour, Southwark, and in 1724 went to St John's College, Cambridge, where six years later he was elected a Fellow. It was after this that he took up the study of medicine, partly in Cambridge and partly in London. In addition to obtaining his degree of Doctor of Medicine in 1739 and later being elected a Fellow of the Royal College of Physicians, in 1749 he was elected a Fellow of the Royal Society. He developed a highly successful consulting practice in London and among his patients were William Cowper, Bishop Warburton and Samuel Johnson. A deeply religious man from his early youth, because of his quiet sincerity and obvious dedication to his work he was held in such high esteem, both by his patients and colleagues, that he had many demands made upon his time and after thirty years in his London practice sought some escape from the rigours of his work by retiring during the summer months to a house in Windsor. He was personal physician to King George III who also invited him to be physician to Queen Charlotte but as his standing was so high he was able to decline this honour as he thought

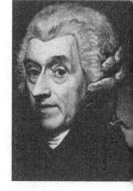

William Heberden
(1710–1801)

it would interfere too much with his other activities. It had been his habit over more than forty years of professional life to review his case notes every month so that he could record in a book any information which he thought might be helpful in the diagnosis and treatment of disease. It was these observations which formed the basis of his famous *Commentaries on the History and Cure of Diseases*, a book which he wrote in Latin after his retirement from practice, at the age of seventy-two. This book, together with an English translation by his son, was published posthumously in 1802. There were numerous editions of the work in both languages as it proved to be one of the most popular medical books in the first part of the nineteenth century. Its contents include his description of chicken pox which was first published in the *Transactions of the Royal College of Physicians of London* in 1768 and his description of the disorder named by him angina pectoris originally reported in the same journal in 1772. His knowledge of the classics led him, in the preface to his book, to liken his life to that of a vestal virgin which, according to Plutarch, is divided into three parts: the first where she learns her professional duties: the second when she practises them: and the third when she teaches them to others. He felt that as he had passed through the first two stages he was willing to devote his last period of life to writing his book so as to teach any of his sons who wished to enter the medical profession.

In chapter 70 entitled 'Pectoris Dolor' he says that, in addition to the pain which may occur in illnesses such as asthma, pleurisy and consumption, the breast is often the seat of pains which, because of their severity and tendency to recur are often distressing but do not affect the general health. Such pains he said which have been called gouty, rheumatic or spasmodic, must be distinguished from another, far more serious disorder which, because of 'the seat of it, and sense of strangling, and anxiety with which it is attended, may make it not improperly be called angina pectoris'. His use of the term angina, derived from the Greek *agkhone* which means strangling, is particularly apposite but 'pectoris' was possibly unfortunate as it might lead some people to imagine that the pain is situated around the left breast. Heberden however was obviously using the word breast synonymously with chest, for later in the chapter he clearly states that it starts across the front of the chest, either at the upper, middle or lower end of the sternum, from where it may spread across the breast into the left arm and at times into the right arm. His description of the classical character of the pain could not be bettered today. He says, 'they who are affected with it are seized while they are walking (more especially if it be uphill and soon after eating) with a painful and most disagreeable sensation in the breast, which seems as if it would extinguish life, if it were to increase or continue; but the moment they stand still all this uneasiness vanishes'. Also he makes particular reference to the case of a man whose constricting pain brought on by exertion and relieved by rest, was entirely classical except that it never affected his chest but was always confined to the left arm alone. This is a variant of angina which is not uncommon but still often leads to diagnostic difficulty and has been described on several occasions since, as if it were an original observation. He recognised that with time the amount of exercise needed to produce angina gets progressively less so that eventually the slightest exertion such as coughing, straining at stool or speaking, will bring on an attack. Also that the condition is aggravated by emotional upsets. Finally, he describes how some of his patients had prolonged pain even when at rest and others suddenly collapsed and died. His observation that males, especially those over the age of fifty, are most liable to this disease is as true today as when he wrote it, but although the number of women with this condition has been increasing in recent years it is surprising that out of nearly a hundred of his patients with angina only three of them were women.

With characteristic modesty in referring to treatment, he said that he had nothing much to advise, pointing out that this was hardly surprising considering that up to then the disease had hardly been recognised or named: nevertheless, with much wisdom, he encouraged the use of quiet, rest, warmth and a judicious use of opium; whilst firmly eschewing bleeding, vomiting and purging, the popular panaceas of his day.

He makes only one reference to the examination of a patient's heart after death from this disease when he says, 'a very skilful anatomist could discover no fault in the heart, in the valves, in the arteries, or neighbouring veins, excepting small rudiments of ossification in the aorta'. It was a remarkable achievement therefore for him to be able to give such a clear and concise account of the disorder from careful observation of his patients and systematic compilation of their notes over the years without knowing anything of the underlying cause of the symptoms.

It is curious that such a shrewd physician did not know more about the pathology of the disease, particularly as he was well aware of the value of post-mortem examinations, for in the preface to his book he remarks, 'an useful addition might have been made to these papers by comparing them ... with the accounts of those who treat of the dissection of morbid bodies; but at my advanced age it would be to no purpose to think of such an undertaking'. Edward Jenner, the Gloucestershire country general practitioner, perhaps best

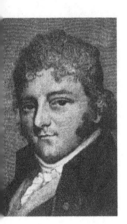

Caleb Parry
(1755–1822)

known for his introduction of smallpox vaccination, and Caleb Parry, the distinguished Bath physician, were before long to become far better informed. This was because both men personally studied the hearts of their patients who had died from angina and being close friends since their grammar school days at Cirencester corresponded with each other on the subject. In one of Jenner's letters to Parry he writes, 'my knife struck something so hard and gritty as to knotch it. I well remember looking up at the ceiling, which was old and crumbling, conceiving that some plaster had fallen down. But on further scrutiny the real cause appeared: the coronaries were become bony canals'. From these and similar observations Jenner could have made his name as the first man to recognise coronary artery disease as the cause of angina but he purposely refrained from publishing his views in order to avoid worrying his revered friend John Hunter, the London surgeon, who in 1773 started to have angina himself. Jenner had had the greatest respect for Hunter since the age of twenty-one when he was sent, after completing two years' apprenticeship to a surgeon in Sodbury near Bristol, to live with Hunter in London for a further two years' study. Hunter, although twenty-one years his senior had much in common with his pupil as in addition to medicine both had a great interest in biology. And when Jenner returned to Gloucestershire they continued a regular correspondence; over the years Hunter obtained many interesting specimens from Jenner, including cuckoos, hedgehogs, eels and salmon spawn. It was in another letter to Parry that Jenner, in discussing the importance of coronary artery narrowing in patients with angina said, 'how much the heart must suffer from their not being able fully to perform their functions ... should it be admitted that this is the cause of the disease I fear the medical world may seek in vain for a remedy, and I am fearful (if Mr H. should admit this to be the cause of the disease) then it may deprive him of the hopes of a recovery'.

Parry, from his own observations, was reaching similar conclusions, and in 1788 read a paper on the subject to the local medical society in Gloucestershire; followed in 1799, six years after Hunter had died from the disease, by the publication of his book entitled *An Inquiry into the Symptoms and Causes of the Syncope Anginosa, commonly called Angina Pectoris; illustrated by Dissections*. In this book he shows that he had a clear understanding that the flow of blood through diseased coronary arteries, although usually sufficient for the requirements of the heart at rest, is totally inadequate when demands were made on it during exertion and that the symptom of angina is the result of this. This concept was further developed by Allan Burns, the Glasgow physician who so regrettably died at the age of thirty-one, probably of a ruptured appendix. In his book,

Observations on Some of the Most Frequent and Important Diseases of the Heart, published in 1809, he likened the effects of stress on a heart with narrowed coronary arteries to those observed in a limb when exercised with a ligature tied round it. And concluded, 'when, therefore, the coronary arteries are ossified every agent capable of increasing the action of the heart, such as exercise, passion and ardent spirits, must be a source of danger'. The adverse influence of emotional disturbance on coronary artery disease may clearly be seen from the detailed account of John Hunter's illness given by his brother-in-law, Everard Home in a preface to Hunter's book, *A Treatise on the Blood, Inflammation and Gunshot Wounds*, published posthumously in this country in 1794 and in Philadelphia in 1796. Home tells us that in the spring of 1773 Hunter was suddenly seized with an excruciating pain in the upper part of the abdomen at 10 o'clock one evening. He thought at first it must be indigestion but while pacing about the room in an endeavour to get relief, by chance caught sight of himself in a mirror and, much to his consternation, saw that his face was so white as to give the appearance of someone dead. Much alarmed he felt for his pulse and finding that he could not detect it in either arm sent for four physicians of whom it is said 'all came but could find no pulse'. The pain lasted for a considerable time and judging from the amount of constitutional disturbance reported must have been a severe attack of coronary thrombosis. The simulation of this attack in its early stage to acute indigestion and Hunter's subsequent suffering from severe flatulence during further attacks is of great interest as it is now recognised that dyspeptic symptoms are not only common in this disease but a constant source of confusion. Further, the description of how his attacks at times were heralded by unpleasant sensations in the face, jaw and throat, was one of the first indications that the feelings of constriction produced by the disease are not confined to the chest and arms alone.

Hunter's angina had the usual relationship to exercise but what was most striking was the frequency with which it was precipitated by emotional distress. Home explained that it was principally anxiety or anger that produced his symptoms whereas occasions which led to feelings of excitement or joy, or times when he was moved by gratitude or compassion even to the point of tears, had no effect. Examples of situations which produced attacks included the hiving of a swarm of bees; anxiety lest an animal should escape before he could get a gun to shoot it; and on one occasion concern that he might have contracted rabies, having cut his finger while performing a post-mortem on a person who had been bitten by a mad dog. It was usually minor irritations such as being kept waiting by a coachman, or a servant failing to carry out his orders, which brought on attacks,

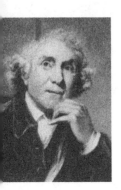

John Hunter
(1728–93)

whereas major crises often had no effect. His realisation that anger had such a powerful influence led him on one occasion to remark that his 'life was in the hands of any rascal who chose to annoy and tease him'. Unfortunately, this prediction was to prove true because it was after an acrimonious hospital committee meeting that he suffered a mortal attack.

Hunter was on the teaching staff of St George's Hospital, London, where it had been customary for the surgeons to share equally the fees obtained from the teaching of students but he rebelled against this method of payment and insisted on it being changed as he found he was doing far more work than the others. He also considered that the bedside teaching given at that time was not adequate and that formal lectures should be introduced similar to those already started at St Bartholomew's Hospital in 1765. His colleagues were so strongly opposed to both these suggestions that the dispute was referred to the General Board of the hospital who appointed a Committee to review all aspects of student teaching. Included among several recommendations of the Committee was that hospital pupils should submit certificates of 'their having been bred up to the profession and of their good behaviour'.

On 16 October, 1793, at a weekly hospital committee meeting, Hunter sought permission for two young men to be admitted to the hospital as pupils under him although they lacked the necessary certificates of being of the required social status. Two of the physicians present violently opposed their admission and in the ensuing quarrel Hunter, finding it difficult to control his anger, abruptly left the meeting. He was no sooner outside than he collapsed and within a few seconds was dead.

There has been much controversy as to the cause of his death, one authority insisting that it was the result of syphilis contracted during an experiment he conducted on himself in May 1767, when he inoculated himself with pus obtained from a patient with venereal disease. Although it is well recognised that syphilis from its effects on the first part of the aorta may seriously damage the cusps of the aortic valve and narrow the mouths of the coronary arteries so that the blood supply to the heart muscle is impaired, with the production of angina, anyone who has read Everard Home's account of the appearances found on post-mortem examination of Hunter's heart can have no doubt that his final illness was not due to syphilis but to an attack of coronary thrombosis. Home described the opaque white areas in the wall of the heart, undoubtedly patches of dead muscle resulting from a thrombus plugging a coronary artery and he later stated that the coronary arteries were like bony tubes which were difficult to divide with a knife, also that the cusps of the aortic valve had undergone similar bony changes. Such changes are quite unlike those of the erosive type of valvular destruction seen in syphilis.

It is now realised that, in coronary artery disease, a degenerative process, which because of its resemblance to porridge is called atheroma, a term derived from the Greek word for gruel, thickens the walls and narrows the lumen of the vessels. Because of this the heart muscle, during exertion, does not obtain sufficient blood for its needs and angina results. At times the blood flowing sluggishly through these arteries suddenly clots, a process known as coronary thrombosis. This obstruction entirely cuts off the blood supply to a part of the heart muscle so that it dies. This, which causes severe anginal type pain, often occurring at rest and accompanied by severe constitutional disturbances, is often fatal. Much confusion occurred among the earlier writers as a clear distinction was not made between angina, the symptom arising from coronary artery narrowing and the more severe type of disease resulting from thrombosis of the blood flowing through the narrowed coronary arteries. There is no doubt that many of the severe cases described by Heberden and Parry were caused by coronary thrombosis as of course was Hunter's death, but the condition was not recognised as a distinct entity until 1876 when Dr Adam Hammer, with considerable clinical acumen, made the diagnosis for the first time at the patient's bedside.

Adam Hammer (1818–78) born in the small town of Mingalsheim, Baden, received his medical education at Heidelberg and then practised in Mannheim until he took part in a general revolution which swept the Continent in 1848. When this failed he emigrated to America where he settled in St Louis. He initiated important reforms in medical education there, and although the teaching institutes he founded did not survive for long he was nevertheless held in high esteem by his colleagues. On 4 May, 1887 he was called into consultation by a doctor who was in doubt as to the diagnosis in a thirty-four-year-old man who was in a state of collapse with an extremely slow pulse. Hammer says in his paper, 'A Case of Thrombotic Occlusion of One of the Coronary Arteries of the Heart', published in 1878, that 'what impressed me particularly about this case and attracted my attention in the highest degree, was the sudden appearance and the steadily progressive course of the collapse'. He considered that this could only be explained by the blood supply to the heart muscle having been suddenly cut off by a thrombotic occlusion of at least one of the coronary arteries. When he put forward this idea his colleague exclaimed, 'I have never heard of such a diagnosis in my whole life', to which Hammer rejoined, 'Nor I, also'. Realising that the patient had only a few hours to live Hammer went to much trouble to obtain permission from the

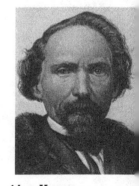

Adam Hammer
(1818–78)

relatives for an autopsy. He said it was difficult at that time in America to obtain such consent and that he often had to purchase it by foregoing his fees or even paying money out of his pocket, adding cynically, 'Before this universal medium even the most subtle misgivings, even the religious ones, soften'. At autopsy, as he had predicted, he found a clotted, jelly-like whitish yellow plug (thrombus) blocking one of the coronary arteries.

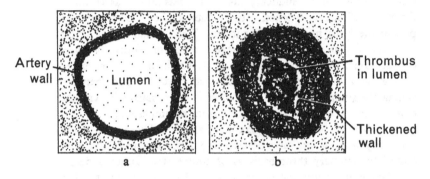

Artery wall — Lumen

Thrombus in lumen

Thickened wall

a   b

Diagrams from photomicrographs of coronary arteries: (a) normal artery: (b) arteriosclerotic artery showing the marked thickening of the wall which results in diminished blood supply to the heart. In addition, in this case, a thrombus has formed in the coronary artery, blocking the circulation

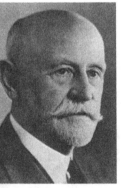

James Herrick (1861–1954)

Since that time it has become recognised that in some adults, particularly in the younger age group, thrombosis of the blood in a coronary artery may occur, as in Hammer's case, without a history of preceding angina because the coronary arteries have only undergone minimal narrowing from degenerative changes in their walls but that in others, usually older people, the thrombosis occurs in vessels already markedly narrowed with a preceding history of effort angina. Further, as with John Hunter, there may be an initial attack of coronary thrombosis, followed by repeated episodes of angina of effort and further attacks of coronary thrombosis. When coronary thrombosis was first recognised as a disease entity such a series of events was not considered possible as it was thought that the coronary arteries were straight tubes without any connecting vessels so that occlusion of an appreciable sized vessel must inevitably be fatal. It was the Chicago physician, Herrick, who early in this century showed that this concept was wrong and that the coronary arteries are connected by numerous small subsidiary vessels which in health remain closed but which are capable of opening up to establish an alternative or collateral circulation when a main vessel becomes blocked.

James Bryan Herrick (1861–1954) was born at Oak Park, Illinois, where his maternal grandfather had settled twenty-eight years earlier, after having travelled westwards in a covered wagon when he emigrated from England to the United States. Herrick graduated in medicine at Rush Medical College in 1888. From that time on his written contributions to medicine were prodigious. It is said that from 1889 to 1935 there were only five individual years in which he did not add to the scientific literature. It was in 1910 that he wrote his first paper on angina pectoris and in 1912 the *Journal of the American Medical Association* published his important paper entitled 'Clinical Features of Sudden Obstruction of the Coronary Arteries'. He said that the idea that recovery from coronary thrombosis was impossible had received support from the experimental work of pathologists including Julius Cohnheim who in 1881 obstructed the coronary arteries in animals by ligatures, with uniformly fatal results. Herrick pointed out that further experimental work by others refuted this belief and drew attention to many of his cases where a coronary thrombosis had been confirmed at autopsy but the patients had lived for several days after the onset of the attack and even in some instances had survived several attacks. He therefore concluded that the symptoms and the outcome in coronary thrombosis must depend on the size of the vessel occluded, the condition of the heart muscle and the ability of the other vessels to maintain an adequate circulation. At the same time he pointed out that a sudden obstruction occurring in a young person with comparatively normal vessels is more likely to lead to sudden death than when there has been gradual narrowing of the lumen of the vessels over a long period with time for an adequate collateral circulation to develop.

It is strange how slow the medical profession was to accept coronary thrombosis as a disease entity and to recognise that its symptoms and signs were the result of death of part of the heart muscle following sudden obstruction of the blood flow through a coronary artery. Although Adam Hammer correctly diagnosed a case of coronary thrombosis in life twenty-two years before the turn of the century it was unfortunate that his report appeared in the *Wiener Medicinische Wochenschrift* where it attracted little or no attention. It was then another thirty-four years before Herrick's paper brought the disease to the notice of doctors in America but in Britain it would seem to have been ignored, possibly because of the preoccupation at that time with the beginning of the First World War. Sir Clifford Allbutt, Professor of Medicine at Cambridge University, published a work in 1915 in which he even rejected the belief that coronary artery disease is the cause of angina. Also Sir James Mackenzie in the third edition

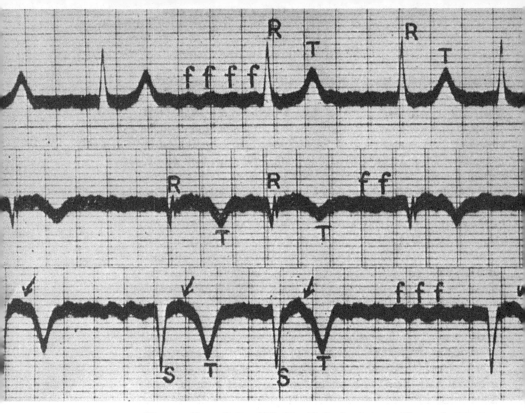

Electrocardiograph in which Harold Pardee in 1925 diagnosed a coronary thrombosis from the characteristic convex curve (indicated by arrows) of the line joining the S and T waves with inversion of the normally upright T wave in the bottom graph

of *Diseases of the Heart*, published in 1913, avoided the term coronary thrombosis and instead referred to angina pectoris as a symptom complex which exhausted the heart muscle.

It was not until the changes produced in the pattern of electro-cardiographic tracings by damaged muscle were identified that coronary thrombosis and its effects on the heart muscle (myocardial infarction) became generally recognised. Sir Thomas Lewis, who had found the electrocardiograph of such great value in the elucidation of disorders of rhythm, during the First World War studied the electrical effects of damage to the ventricles. The changes in the T wave of the electrocardiograph associated with sudden obstruction of a coronary artery received brief mention from Herrick in 1919. Credit for the detailed description of these changes, however, must be given to Harold Pardee of New York who in 1920 described the electrocardiographic findings in a patient four hours after the onset of the attack and at regular intervals after. He showed that at an early stage the line joining the Q, R, S, complex to the beginning of the T wave instead of being straight starts from near the top of the R wave to form a downwards concave curve, now known as Pardee's curve, and in 1925 pointed out that at a later stage it returns to the base line but the T wave instead of being upright becomes deeply inverted. The clinical diagnosis in Britain became more frequent once Sir John Parkinson and D. E. Bedford, in 1926, reported a large series of cases showing these typical electrocardiographic changes. Since then the number of diagnosed cases has increased enormously partly because of physicians' greater awareness but also because of an undoubted rise in the incidence of the disease. The cause of this has been the subject of much speculation.

It was Sir William Osler, when Professor of Medicine at Oxford, who first emphasised that certain types of individual appear to have an increased susceptibility to coronary artery disease because of hereditary or environmental factors. In the second of his two lectures on angina pectoris to the Royal College of Physicians in 1910 he said he had found the disease to be far more prevalent among the upper classes who consulted him in his private practice than among the poorer people he attended in hospital. He thought this was surprising considering that the poor are constantly subjected to worry and hard work and considered that possibly certain families with a hereditary predisposition developed a special strain of tissue with a particular liability to react 'anginally'. In support of this he noted that it was not uncommon for it to occur in successive generations of the same family. His wide clinical experience and highly developed powers of perception led him to recognise that people with certain psychological and physical attributes are especially prone to the disease. He said, 'It is not the delicate neurotic person who is prone to angina, but the robust, the vigorous in mind and body, the keen and ambitious man, the indicator of whose engines is always at "full speed ahead"', an apt description of what today would be described as the muscular extroverted ambitious type, whose sudden unexpected death in middle life is now so distressingly common.

Since Osler's time the personal observations of this sagacious physician have been amplified and augmented by numerous large, long-term prospective population surveys. Most of these have been American. They include the studies at the National Heart Institute at Framingham, Mass., where 5,127 symptom-free people have been followed for more than twelve years and the constitutional and environmental factors in the 125 men and 61 women who developed coronary artery disease during this period have been compared with the remainder. A similar study was undertaken in the ten-year Survey at the Albany, New York, Cardiovascular Health Centre. In Chicago, since the autumn of 1957, members of the University of Illinois College of Medicine have conducted a long-term study of workers at the Western Electric Company; and in Minnesota, since

1948 there has been a fifteen-year study of coronary artery disease arising in business and professional men. In Britain there have been, up to now, few reports of long-term prospective studies. An important recent one was conducted by the Medical Research Council's Social Medicine Research Unit at the London Hospital in which 667 middle-aged London bus men were followed for five years. These studies, together with others, have led to the conclusion that there are multiple interrelated causes for coronary artery disease rather than any single predominant one. The factors associated with a high incidence of the disease include a raised blood pressure: an increased amount of cholesterol in the blood: excessive cigarette smoking and obesity. The development of some of these is governed by a hereditary predisposition.

The adverse effect of a persistently raised blood pressure has been confirmed by reports both in Britain and America. In Britain the value of blood pressure readings in predicting the future onset of coronary artery disease was confirmed by a long-term survey of a Welsh community published in 1959. And by a report in 1966 of a medico-actuarial investigation which showed that the level of blood pressure at initial examinations is related to the risk of subsequent death from coronary artery disease. Hypertension, however, is not essential for the production of coronary artery disease, it is present in only about 50 per cent of men and about 75 per cent of women with this disorder. Its importance obviously becomes greater when present with other factors but, like all causes of this disease, is not necessarily of significance by itself. In Japan, although it is common to find high levels of blood pressure, because other factors are absent, coronary artery disease is rare. In the American Framingham Survey elevation of blood pressure was associated with a twofold increase in the risk of coronary artery disease in males and sixfold in females and for every individual the chance of developing the disease increased proportionally with the height of the blood pressure. In the English study of London Transport bus drivers and conductors the level of the blood pressure was one of the two factors which stood out most clearly as having an important predictive value.

Cigarette smoking has been found in all surveys to be a predominant factor and may well prove to be one of the outstanding causes of the alarming increase in cases of coronary artery disease in the Western world during recent years. It is tragic that the warnings about the dangers of smoking issued by the Royal College of Physicians of London and the Surgeon-General in Washington have largely been disregarded by the public. The data from the Framingham Survey, when studied in combination with that from Albany, New York, and published in 1962, based on a study of 4,120 men, showed that heavy cigarette smoking led to a threefold increase in incidence of coronary artery disease. The Survey at the Chicago Western Electric Company showed a similar high significant association with the smoking of cigarettes but not of pipe tobacco or cigars. A similar relationship has been noted by Doll and Hill in their ten years' observation of British doctors which included a study of their mortality from coronary thrombosis in relation to smoking. Their report, published in 1966, shows that death from coronary artery disease increases with the number of cigarettes smoked daily and that amongst smokers of twenty-five cigarettes or more a day the age-adjusted death rate for coronary artery disease was nearly eight times that of non-smokers. The American report, *The Health Consequences of Smoking*, published in 1967 by the Surgeon-General's Advisory Committee and based on five very large prospective mortality studies confirms that cigarette smokers have substantially higher death rates from coronary artery disease than do non-smokers; that cigarette smoking markedly increases the individual's susceptibility to earlier death from the disease; and confirms that mortality rates are proportional to cigarette consumption. It was found that the mortality rate for coronary thrombosis for smokers between the ages of forty-five and fifty-four who smoked ten or more cigarettes a day is three times as great for men and twice as great for women, as compared with non-smokers. It has been suggested that the adverse effect of cigarette smoking is possibly because it stimulates the secretion of epinephrine and nor-epinephrine from the adrenal glands which appear to act, not by constricting the coronary arteries themselves but by increasing the heart rate and raising the blood pressure so as to put an extra load on the heart.

Actuarial surveys in Britain have shown that obesity is a significant risk when the body weight is more than 20 per cent above the normal for the individual; a finding confirmed by similar large-scale studies published by the American Society of Actuaries. Also the records of life assurance companies show that the mortality from coronary artery disease is 40 per cent higher in fat people than among the normal population and that obesity is particularly dangerous when accompanied by a high blood pressure.

The importance of obesity as a factor predisposing to this disease leads to a consideration of the dietetic habits of those at risk. There is no doubt that Western civilisation is addicted to food and that the majority of people overeat. There is much controversy at the moment however as to the relative importance of excess fat or sugar in the diet and at the same time there is growing awareness of the importance of inherited errors in the metabolism of these substances.

The evidence about fats is particularly confusing; a marked fall in degenerative disease of the arteries was noted in Germany immediately after the First World War at a time when the fat content of the diet was low; similarly, there was a decrease in the incidence of arterial degeneration in Norway and other occupied countries during the Second World War, thought to be due to a great reduction in the fat content of the diet. It is difficult to understand however how a sudden and temporary fall in the fat content of the diet of a community could effect degenerative changes in arteries which are known to take very long periods to develop. There is no doubt that the incidence of coronary artery disease increased markedly in Jews when they left the Yemen, where their diet was low in fat, and emigrated to Israel where the diet is rich in fat. But it is difficult to assess the importance of this change as there was a concomitant increase in the sugar intake which, as will be discussed later, may have been of importance. A study of inhabitants in Cape Town showed that whereas coronary artery disease is rare amongst Bantus whose fat intake is low, it is fairly common amongst negroes with a moderate amount of fat in their diet and very prevalent amongst the Europeans whose diet is similar to that of Europeans living in England and America. Again there are difficulties however in drawing conclusions because the low fat diet of the Bantu does not protect him from degenerative arterial changes in the brain, the incidence of which is as high as amongst the Europeans; it is possible therefore that the Bantus' protection from coronary artery disease may be more readily attributed to other factors such as greater physical exertion and less cigarette smoking. Among the Japanese living in Japan the disease is rare. At first sight this might seem to be an example of hereditary protection until it is realised that it occurs fairly often in the Japanese in Hawaii and is as common in the second-generation Japanese in Los Angeles as it is in the white population there. The influence of heredity undoubtedly plays a part in the aetiology of this disease but this is an example where its incidence in one race has altered remarkably with changes in diet, the fat intake in America being about three times that in Japan. It has been suggested that it is the gradual increase in the fat content of the American nation's diet during this century which has coincided with the increased incidence of coronary artery disease. The blood content of cholesterol, a substance found in animal fats but not usually in vegetable fats, is now used as an index of susceptibility to coronary artery disease. When blood cholesterol studies were done in Israel it was found that the cholesterol content of those recently arrived from the Yemen was significantly lower than in those who had lived in Israel for many years while at the same time much higher levels were found among recent immigrants from western Europe. These differences are considered to correlate with the varying fat intake and to be a reflection of the varying liability to coronary artery disease in these three groups. Similarly, American Seventh Day Adventists, whose diet contains much less animal fat than the average American, have a substantially lower cholesterol level and, although not necessarily directly because of this, have less coronary artery disease.

The cholesterol blood level is not always directly related to fat intake as it is also affected by other factors such as cigarette smoking which may possibly raise the level, emotional stress, which is thought to raise it, exercise which is known to lower it, and inherited errors of metabolism which also influence it. In the important long-term surveys in Albany, Framingham and Chicago, in all of which a high serum cholesterol level was found to be an adverse prognostic factor, there was no conclusive evidence that the plasma cholesterol of any individual was related to the dietary intake of fats.

There are certain families in which, because of an inherited error of metabolism, all members have a high serum cholesterol and who are also particularly prone to develop coronary artery disease often in early adult life. The susceptibility to coronary artery disease however is not necessarily directly due to this high plasma cholesterol level because there is no good evidence that lowering it with various drugs such as clofibrate alters the incidence of coronary occlusive disease in these patients.

There is increasingly strong evidence that excessive sugar in the diet and disturbance of the metabolism of sugar in the body plays an important part. Professor Yudkin in England has claimed that the rise in mortality from degenerative heart disease has corresponded more closely with the national increase in the consumption of refined sugar than that of any other constituent of the diet, including fats. It is difficult to explain however on this hypothesis why the mortality among young men has increased so markedly as compared with women since the First World War as the intake of sugar by men is not appreciably higher. Neither does it explain the increased incidence in recent years of sudden heart attacks among the population in the lower-income groups who, for economic reasons have always had a diet with a preponderance of starches. There is however clear evidence that coronary artery disease occurs commonly in people whose metabolism of sugar is faulty. For a long time it has been known that diabetics are particularly prone to arterial degenerative changes. Now it is realised that not only they, but also people who do not suffer from the disease themselves, but have a history of diabetes in other members of their family, develop arterial disorders frequently and at an early age; further, that when such young people with coronary artery disease who have not overt diabetes but who have a family history of the disease, are subjected to serial blood sugar studies, nearly 50 per cent of them are found to show evidence of a disturbed metabolism. There is thus good evidence that families with a genetic liability to disorders of sugar metabolism are particularly liable to the early development of arterial degenerative diseases. As diabetes mellitus often has an insidious onset blood sugar estimations have been carried out on apparently fit people in large community surveys. These include the one conducted by Epstein and others in Tecumseh, Michigan, and also one by the Department of Medical Statistics and Epidemiology at the London School of Hygiene and Tropical Medicine in conjunction with the Department of Medicine at Guy's Hospital, in a population at Bedford, England. Both reports, published in 1965, show that there is a large amount of unsuspected diabetes in a community and also an appreciable number of people who, although not true diabetics, have blood sugar tests which show minor but definite abnormalities. Also, that in both these groups there is a far higher incidence of symptoms from arterial degeneration and electrocardiographic evidence of coronary artery disease, than in the normal population.

Coronary artery disease is much more frequent among males than females but this predominance does not exist among diabetics and is less evident in hypertensives and in those over the age of sixty. Both men and women have the hormone oestrogen in their bodies but it is the larger quantity of this in women which is thought to protect them from coronary artery disease.

As Osler observed, there does seem to be a definite type of person whose physical and psychological characteristics are associated with susceptibility to coronary artery disease. The physical characteristics of men prone to this disorder are predominant 'maleness, muscularity and compactness'. The psychological characteristics are more difficult to define. The disease has generally been thought to be more common in ambitious executive types, fired by competitive drive and subjected to worry and responsibility: but in a disease which is now so widespread and which affects so many people throughout all the various strata of society it is difficult to distinguish a clear-cut personality type. Recent studies in large American organisations such as the Bell Telephone and the Dupont companies showed that the death rate from coronary artery disease was in fact lower in executives than in clerks.

Perhaps the most intriguing example of what has been considered to be the effect of social competitive stress has been afforded by a study of degenerative heart disease in mammals at the Zoological Gardens in Philadelphia. Accurate autopsy records of these animals are available from 1901 and deaths from this cause were unknown until recent years when there has been an epidemic. The diet has been of high quality and unchanged in character since 1935 but five years before coronary artery disease started to occur a major change in policy in the housing and grouping of the animals took place and it is thought that the emotional stresses associated with this precipitated the epidemic. It is difficult to evaluate the effects of emotional stress because as with all other factors there is always a large number of other concurrent influences at work. The low incidence of coronary thrombosis among those who, while subjected to all the rigours of war, were at the same time kept in states of semi-starvation, is strongly against nervous stress having a primary role. There seems no doubt however that stress when combined with other factors may be important and as John Hunter found, an acute emotional crisis may not uncommonly precipitate anginal pain. The protective value of regular exercise seems to be well substantiated. This may be associated with its effect of lowering the level of cholesterol in the blood. This biochemical change in response to exertion was thought to have been an important factor in the lower incidence of coronary artery disease amongst bus conductors as compared with bus drivers in the study of London Transport employees. A study published in 1966 of the records of 40,000 students at the universities of Pennsylvania and Harvard showed that a high proportion of men who ultimately died from coronary artery disease did not take part in organised games when at college. This group also, however, amongst other factors, had an increased incidence of emotional disorders and it is studies like this that clearly demonstrate the difficulty of evaluating the significance of any one factor.

The ideal, therefore, is to avoid emotional stress and to take plenty of exercise but that neither of these is as important as avoiding dietary excess may be seen from a study of an unfortunate nomadic tribe in North Kenya whose people live a carefree, physically strenuous life but who, because of a diet very rich in fat, have high levels of plasma cholesterol and a high incidence of coronary artery disease.

It may therefore be seen from this discussion that the situation is complex but sufficient adverse factors have been identified to allow some remarkably accurate predictive studies to be made. Perhaps the two most important factors are an abnormally high blood pressure and a raised serum cholesterol level. It was these which were found to be of most significance in the London Transport survey. Also, an American study published in 1961 showed that when they were both present in the same individual, together with evidence of cardiac enlargement, it was found that 500 out of 1,000 men aged forty to fifty-nine, experienced coronary artery disease within a six-year period of observation whereas the disease only developed in 36 out of

200 men without these three findings. Another report in 1964 showed that when 600 New York executives were analysed with respect to blood pressure, serum cholesterol, phospholipid and uric acid levels, height, body build, age and causes of death in parents and siblings, 39 were selected as 'prone to coronary heart disease'. They were then followed up over a period of five years during which time 38 of them developed the condition.

Western civilisation is in the midst of an epidemic of coronary artery disease. In England it caused the death of 48 people out of every million living in 1926, 148 in 1936, 473 in 1939, 1,392 in 1953 and by 1963 the number had increased by approximately half as many again. Although there are many operative factors it would seem that some of the most important are related to long-term over-nutrition. It is a striking commentary on the present disturbing times to reflect that one-half of the world is threatened with death from starvation whilst the other half is killing itself from dietary over-indulgence. This epidemic is now affecting far more women than in the past and in men, although the disease has for a long time been prevalent from middle age upwards, it is now not uncommonly occurring in those under forty. It is alarming to learn that when young Americans with an average age of twenty-two, killed in battle in the Korean War, had their hearts examined, nearly 80 per cent of them already showed evidence of degenerative changes in the coronary arteries. It would seem therefore that preventive measures must start in childhood by parents ceasing to over-feed their children and in later life by adults avoiding over-indulgence in food and cigarettes and for people of all ages to take plenty of exercise.

13

Preventing and combating 'heart attacks'

THE first step in the treatment of angina is to ascertain its cause. By the end of the nineteenth century it was known that the common cause is narrowing of the coronary arteries from degenerative changes in the walls of those vessels; also that it may be caused by narrowing of the mouths of the coronary arteries by syphilitic disease in the wall of the aorta; or by stenosis of the aortic valve reducing the flow of blood through them. It was not however until 1918 that Herrick and his colleague Nuzum showed that in addition angina may occur when the heart muscle is deprived of oxygen because of severe anaemia.

Anginal pain was relieved in Heberden's time by laudanum, a preparation of opium, or by alcoholic stimulants such as brandy, and in later years by the inhalation of anaesthetic substances such as ether and chloroform. The introduction of amyl nitrite by Lauder Brunton in 1867 was a great advance.

Lauder Brunton (1844–1916) the youngest son of a farmer at Bowden, Roxburghshire, Scotland, studied medicine at the University of Edinburgh where he qualified in 1866. It was whilst serving as a house physician to the Professor of Medicine at Edinburgh University that he discovered the beneficial effects of amyl nitrite. In addition to his routine clinical duties Brunton was engaged at that time in a study of the effects of drugs on the blood pressure, using Marey's sphygmograph, which had been invented four years previously. With this instrument Brunton studied the effect of digitalis on his own blood pressure and also observed the elevation in blood pressure which occurs when a person has an attack of angina. He further showed that the drug amyl nitrite lowered this raised pressure and in so doing reduced the load on the heart and abolished the pain; thus he not only discovered a valuable drug but also gave an ingenious explanation of the mechanism of its action. Some years later experiments on the hearts of healthy animals showed that the direct application of nitrites to coronary arteries caused the muscle

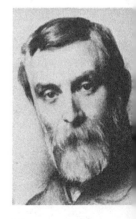

Sir Thomas Lauder Brunton (1844–1916)

in their walls to relax so that the blood flow through them was increased. It was then taught that this must be the obvious mode of action in angina and amyl nitrite, together with other nitrites later introduced were classified as coronary artery dilators. A cursory examination of vessels sufficiently diseased as to cause angina is enough to show that they are extremely rigid without much ability to dilate and in any case the oxygen lack which accompanies this condition is such a powerful stimulant to any possible dilatation that the administration of drugs is extremely unlikely to increase this. Modern pharmacologists have therefore reverted to the original teaching of Brunton and accept that the beneficial effect of these drugs is not a direct one on the coronary arteries but is achieved by their effect of lowering the blood pressure.

Brunton's epoch-making discovery in his first year as a medical practitioner marked the beginning of a brilliant career. He left Edinburgh for London in 1870 when he became a lecturer in pharmacology at the Middlesex Hospital and a year later was appointed to the teaching staff of St Bartholomew's Hospital where he remained until his retirement in 1904. His particular interests were physiology and pharmacology, knowledge of which he advanced by painstaking experiments on himself, his students, and animals. His lectures at St Bartholomew's Hospital on the use of drugs based on his study of their action in the body were so revolutionary that they were always crowded, not only by his own pupils but by students and teachers from other schools. At the early age of thirty he was elected a Fellow of the Royal Society in recognition of his work on the physiology of digestion, the chemical composition of blood, the action of digitalis and of mercury. He made numerous contributions to medical literature and from time to time collected them together and reprinted them in book form. In 1907 he published his *Collected Papers on Circulation and Respiration*, amongst which is his classic 'On the use of Nitrite of Amyl in Angina Pectoris', first published in the *Lancet* in 1867. In this paper Brunton pointed out that amyl nitrite, first discovered by Balard, was subjected to clinical investigation by Guthrie who noticed that it caused flushing of the face, throbbing of the arteries in the neck, and increased the speed of the heart, and because of this recommended it as a stimulant in cases of drowning, suffocation and fainting.

Little practical use however was made of this drug until Dr Arthur Gamgee, in an unpublished series of experiments, many of which Brunton witnessed, showed that it lowers the arterial tension both in animals and man. It was these observations, Brunton said, that led him to try its effect in angina. He explained that he had observed that whereas brandy is not particularly helpful in controlling this type of pain and that chloroform inhaled in sufficient quantities as to produce partial stupefaction only gave temporary relief, that small bleedings of three or four ounces whether by cupping or venesection were always effective. It was because he thought this procedure must have its effect by lowering the arterial tension that he was prompted to try the effect of amyl nitrite. At first he used it by getting the patient to inhale five to ten drops of the drug which he poured on to a cloth and was delighted to find that within a minute and simultaneously with flushing of the face and lowering of the blood pressure, the chest pain disappeared. Later, the drug, which is an inflammable volatile liquid, was dispensed in glass capsules which, when broken between finger and thumb, was inhaled through the open mouth. Its action when administered in this manner is immediate and effective but its characteristic smell makes the patient conspicuous and it also produces a severe throbbing headache. It was nevertheless a great advance as it was the first effective drug in the treatment of angina.

Brunton's outstanding merit was recognised by numerous honours bestowed on him by learned societies not only in this country but in America, France and Russia, where he was made a member of the Imperial Military Academy of Medicine of St Petersburg. He received a knighthood in 1900 and was created a baronet in 1908.

The next step following the discovery of amyl nitrite was the introduction of nitroglycerin by William Murrell in 1879 for use in the treatment of angina. William Murrell (1853–1912) like Lauder Brunton, took a particular interest in the scientific investigation of the action of drugs. This was unusual among the physicians of his time on the staff of teaching hospitals who not only made no reference to pharmacology in their teaching but discouraged research on the subject and even demonstrated their apathy by not bothering with the details of prescribing drugs which they left to their house physicians. Murrell was fortunate because at an early stage in his career he worked with Sidney Ringer, at a time when this physiologist was conducting extensive experiments on the effect of drugs on living animal tissues. Inspired by the importance of this work Murrell devoted the rest of his life to a study of therapeutics undeterred by, but bitterly disappointed at, the discouraging attitude of his colleagues. His important paper, 'Nitroglycerin as a Remedy for Angina Pectoris', was published in the *Lancet* in 1879 when he was still only twenty-six years of age and a lecturer in physiology at the Westminster Hospital.

The drug had given rise to interest long before this, for when Murrell was still only a small child a certain Mr A. G. Field of Brighton reported in the columns of the *Medical Times and Gazette* the various unpleasant effects nitroglycerin had when he took it himself and also when administered to his patients, but also its efficacy in the treatment of neuralgic pain. He said that after taking only two drops of a 1 per cent solution of nitroglycerin in alcohol he experienced temporary mental confusion, with noises in the ears like steam escaping from a kettle, nausea, mental and physical exhaustion which lasted for half an hour, together with a headache which lasted for several hours. In spite of these unpleasant effects he tried to persuade a friend to take a dose but it is said that that gentleman developed such alarming symptoms after only licking the cork of the bottle that he would have no more to do with the substance. Undeterred by this Field placed a half drop of the solution on the tongue of a patient suffering from toothache whereupon she fainted, but on recovering was relieved to find that although she had a throbbing headache the pain had gone. Another patient accidentally swallowed a piece of lint which Field had soaked in a solution of nitroglycerin and applied to a decayed tooth. This lady also lost consciousness for a few minutes but on recovery, in spite of a headache, was gratified to find that the pain in her tooth had disappeared. It was from these and other experiences that Field concluded that the drug was of therapeutic value and his report induced other medical men to try the effect of the drug for themselves. Dr George Harley of University College, having obtained some nitroglycerin of the same strength as that used by Field, did no more at first than cautiously lick the cork of the bottle: as this produced only a transitory feeling of fullness in his head and possibly slight tightness about the throat, symptoms which he thought may well have been only due to imagination, he took five drops of the solution and then, finding this had no effect, a further ten drops. Although he felt nothing untoward he was by this time frightened in case he had taken too much and probably because of this his heart began to thump: when, however, he found that he was left with no more than a residual headache he gave much larger doses to two medical friends but again without any ill effects. Encouraged by this he took some pure nitroglycerin in a dose equivalent to one hundred drops of the initial dilute solution and subsequently gave himself and other people twice as much without experiencing anything more troublesome than a fast pulse and some throbbing in the head.

Another person who was sceptical about the potency of the drug was Dr Fuller of St George's Hospital who, having written disparagingly about it, received a personal visit from Mr Field. Field persuaded him to take the same dose as had caused himself so much discomfort but was much surprised to find this dose had little effect on Dr Fuller, other than a slight headache. As headache seems to have been a constant side effect with this substance it is surprising to learn that on that same day Field administered it to a hospital patient suffering with migraine. He must have initially regretted this because the patient broke out into a profuse sweat and fainted. After however being revived with ammonia he found his headache was so much improved that he was able to sleep and Field, encouraged by this apparent success, continued to administer it to several other people.

Murrell, twenty years later, on looking back over some past journals, came across the reports of this interesting controversy and thinking it strange that people should have experienced such widely differing effects from the drug, decided, somewhat courageously, to try it on himself. One afternoon, while holding an out-patient clinic, he suddenly remembered that the bottle containing the solution he had obtained for this purpose was in his pocket, and in his eagerness to try its effects, straightway applied the moistened cork to his tongue. He must quickly have regretted this impulse for he says that he experienced a violent pulsation in his head and 'Mr Field's observations rose considerably in my estimation'. Before long his heart beat rapidly and his pulse was so forceful that it made his hands jerk violently. He began to wish that he had chosen a more opportune time to conduct his experiment for he was concerned lest his patients, noticing his distress, might think he was ill or intoxicated. Provided he kept quiet he found the symptoms bearable but they became so marked on exertion that he resolved not to percuss his patients' chest but to restrict his activities to the application of a stethoscope. The movement however of bending down to listen to a chest caused an almost intolerable pounding in his head and although this quickly abated he was left with a throbbing headache for the rest of the afternoon. He was certain that his symptoms were not due to imagination or nervousness although he was very surprised to find himself so severely affected after having read about Dr Harley's reassuring experiences. The incident did not deter him, for following this he took the drug about forty times but with the precaution of administering it only in some place where he could sit quietly and avoid the aggravating effects of exertion. Even so he found that the effect on his pulse was so marked that its forceful beating jerked his whole body and with ingenuity he measured the degree of pulsation by holding a looking-glass in his hand and throwing the reflection into a dark corner of the room.

In trying to correlate the effects of this drug on himself and the varying results produced on others, he came to the conclusion that there must be individual differences of susceptibility and thus persuaded several people, including some of his personal friends, to try its effect. He was able to observe its action in twelve men and twenty-three women. As might be expected he found that women and debilitated men were more easily affected by it. Everyone however, even the most robust men, seemed to have had quite severe untoward side effects but several of them claimed relief from long-standing neuralgia pains. Their fortitude seems remarkable and one friend whom he persuaded to continue to take four drops of the solution every four hours, in spite of the fact that it gave him a throbbing headache was convinced that it relieved him of an old-standing facial neuralgia. One young man, given nitroglycerin in mistake for phosphorus, found that after each dose the pulsation set up in his body was so severe and prolonged and accompanied by an intense burning and flushing of his face and feeling of general exhaustion that he was frightened. It might be thought that he would have desisted, even after the first dose, but such must have been his faith in his medical adviser that he persevered until quite a large amount had been taken. A woman was ordered to take single drop doses of the 1 per cent solution every four hours. As this had no effect the dose was gradually increased so that after five weeks she was taking ten times the amount; each dose then made her faint, on one occasion for ten minutes, followed by violent trembling and vomiting. Her husband and friends were greatly alarmed but such is the power of persuasion and faith that she herself considered that on the whole it had done her good.

Unpleasant though these side effects must have been Murrell fortunately saw in them a similarity to those produced by amyl nitrite. He concluded that the drug therefore might be of use in the treatment of angina pectoris and set about comparing the effect of the two drugs with the help of a sphygmograph. His paper reporting the action of nitroglycerin in the treatment of angina pectoris was based on the effect it had on three patients with this condition, whom he had seen in the previous nine months. He administered it as a 1 per cent nitroglycerin solution in a half ounce of water three times a day and found that this reduced the number of attacks; also that it afforded relief when taken during an episode of pain.

Nitroglycerin, or glyceryl trinitrate as it is now usually called, is an oily liquid which although non-inflammable explodes on concussion with a force greater than that of gunpowder. Pharmacists for many years have therefore mixed it with inert substances and dispensed it in tablets. In this form it is safe and stable, whilst retaining its potency for a much longer time than the liquid preparation which quickly evaporates. Its efficacy in the relief of angina was soon established and it remains the drug of choice to this day.

The treatment of coronary thrombosis resolves itself into the relief of pain with morphine or other similar powerful analgesics, bed-rest, the maintenance of an adequate blood pressure, the use of drugs such as digitalis when the muscle of the heart fails as a pump, and the use of this and other drugs to combat any serious disorders of rhythm which may arise. The use of drugs known as anticoagulants in an effort to influence the clotting process responsible for the thrombosis has been disappointing. Heparin, a drug discovered by a medical student, J. McClean in 1916 at the Johns Hopkins Medical School in America is perhaps the best. McClean was studying the clot-promoting activity of organic lipoid substances known as phosphatides when to his surprise he found that a liver extract prolonged the clotting time of blood. Further investigation showed that the active principle was a mucopolysaccharide present in many organs but as he happened to isolate it from liver, the Latin name for which is *hepar*, he called it heparin. Heparin, now prepared commercially from ox-lung, is ineffective when given by mouth but has a powerful effect when given into a vein. Injections have to be repeated every four to six hours, so it is only suitable for treatment in hospital and on a short-term basis. Another group of anticoagulant drugs, the coumarins, may be given by mouth and therefore are more suitable for prolonged use but, as there is a time lag before they exert their effect, heparin is usually given in addition for the first forty-eight hours. The discovery of the coumarins dates back to the early 1920s when a new and strange disease in cows began to trouble farmers in North America. Cattle were found to have copious haemorrhages, sometimes occurring spontaneously and sometimes after injury, so that cows bled to death after they had been de-horned and young bulls did the same after castration. F. W. Schofield, a veterinary pathologist, described the disease in the *Journal of the American Veterinary Medical Association* in 1924. A new fodder crop known as sweet clover had recently been introduced and Schofield observed that it was cattle fed on this foodstuff when it was mouldy, which bled. By experimental feeding of rabbits he confirmed that it was some toxic substance in this mouldy sweet clover which was the cause. This report led to much research, culminating in the isolation of the active principle, dicoumarol, by the American chemist Link, in 1941. Coumarins are present in many plants, give new-mown hay and grass their characteristic smell, and are much used in the perfume industry. Their effect in the body when given in small doses is to prevent the clotting of blood without causing uncontrollable bleeding and because of this have been in use for some years in the treatment of coronary thrombosis. Unfortunately, once a clot has already formed in a coronary artery there is no evidence that anticoagulant drugs prevent its extension along the length of the vessel and their use for this purpose has been disappointing. However, these drugs are usefully employed during the first few weeks after the event as they help to prevent clots from forming on the damaged wall of the affected ventricle and in the veins of the legs; also they prevent any clots which might form from fragmenting. This is very important as the movement of pieces of clot from one place to another such as from the left ventricle to the brain, is always serious and from the leg veins to the lungs may be fatal. At first it was thought that anticoagulants might be helpful on a long-term basis for the prevention of further episodes of clotting in the coronary arteries but it has been very difficult to obtain conclusive evidence that this occurs. The British Medical Research Council's report in 1964 stated that the prophylactic use of these drugs for one to two years might cause a slight benefit for men under fifty-five years, but is not of any value for older men or for women in any age group. Since the isolation of dicoumarin in 1941, several other drugs with certain advantages over the parent substance, have been synthesised, phenindione (Dindevan) is now widely used as well as warfarin (Marevan) which has also become popular as a rat poison!

Recently there have been certain other advances in the treatment of coronary thrombosis particularly in the management of disorders of the heart's rate and rhythm in this condition and, most dramatic of all, the introduction of techniques which now makes it possible in certain cases to save a patient's life after his heart has stopped beating. It might be assumed that cardiac arrest would always be fatal but surgeons, for some years now, have known that when for one reason or another a heart stops beating during an operation it is occasionally possible to revive it by massaging it with the hand, also that an electric shock applied directly to the heart is capable of stopping a heart, restoring its action, or changing the rhythm of its beats. In the last decade, by an extension of these measures, applied externally through the intact chest wall, it has sometimes been found possible to counteract cardiac arrest following a coronary thrombosis. This has been shown only to be successful, however, if the damage to the heart muscle is not already too severe and provided skilled resuscitation is started within minutes. Credit for the remarkable discovery that the heart can be effectively 'massaged' from outside the chest must be given to Kouwenhoven, Jude and Knickerbocker who in 1962, in the *Journal of the American Medical Association*, reported that it was possible, by exerting strong pressure on the chest wall to compress the heart between the sternum and the spine and that by repeating the procedure rhythmically about eighty times a minute, to restore an adequate circulation of blood to the body, provided that at the same time respiration is maintained artificially by mouth to mouth breathing. These two first-aid manœuvres are now taught to all nurses so that they can be initiated without any delay and continued until a team of doctors can take over. An anaesthetist continues the artificial respiration of the patient by using a mechanical respirator attached to a tube placed in the trachea; while another doctor inserts a needle into a vein in order to set up a sodium bicarbonate transfusion to correct the chemical changes which take place in the blood; a third continues external massage. While all this is taking place an electrocardiograph is recorded, the tracing by this time may show that there is still no evidence of spontaneous action of the heart, or that the cardiac massage has been successful in restoring it to a normal action, or that there is a peculiar ineffectual writhing movement of the ventricles known as ventricular fibrillation. This disorder of rhythm is similar to atrial fibrillation but far more dangerous because if left unchecked the heart cannot maintain an adequate circulation and death is inevitable. Fortunately, the recent invention of a special electrical apparatus has made it possible to convert this dangerous disorder of rhythm back to normal by a powerful electric shock delivered to the heart through two electrodes placed on the chest wall. From this brief account it may be readily appreciated that any potentially successful attempt at cardiac resuscitation requires much expensive apparatus and a team of skilled doctors and nurses immediately available. This has led in recent years to the setting up of special intensive coronary care units in the larger hospitals: such units are equipped with special electrocardiographic monitors which, when attached to a patient, record on a screen the wave pattern produced by the electrical impulses arising from the heart. This enables doctors and nurses at a glance to observe the rate and rhythm of the heart so that immediate action may be taken if the heart suddenly stops or beats too slowly or too fast, especially if it becomes irregular with multiple extra beats or if the ventricles start to fibrillate.

Most people who suffer a serious coronary thrombosis do so outside hospital and not only may the stress and anxiety of an ambulance journey to hospital aggravate their condition but many of them need the skilled care of a trained team immediately. It is for this reason that in some areas, as an experiment, a mobile team has been formed, ready at a moment's notice to go from the hospital to the patient. This idea is not new; in Russia such emergency arrangements have existed in large cities for the past ten years. It is however very expensive in terms of medical manpower and certainly the present staffing of district hospitals in Britain would have to be much increased in order to provide this service.

The prevention of coronary thrombosis is certainly far more

rewarding than the treatment: although many factors such as those associated with inherited predisposition are unavoidable there are two particularly important steps which can be taken by everyone. These are the avoidance of excessive cigarette smoking and obesity. Commercial enterprise has prospered through the sale of expensive preparations of food said to be particularly suited to people liable to coronary artery disease but all that matters is that the diet should be sufficiently low in calories to avoid overweight. Obesity has of course always been common but never considered anything more than an inconvenience until recent years when its close association with the high incidence of coronary artery disease has been recognised. It is unfortunate that carbohydrates are cheap to buy and attractive to eat whereas protein is expensive and, by itself, uninteresting. The pleasure of food and its comforting effect in times of stress makes it very difficult for many people to accept the discipline of keeping their weight within proper limits especially as the years advance, and for this reason there has always been the wish to find some other method of doing it such as exercise and the taking of drugs. Although regular exercise is essential for health, unfortunately it has little effect on weight and, indeed, by increasing the appetite, often has the opposite effect. There are also no safe and effective drugs for this purpose. Thyroid, much in vogue for many years, has no effect except when there is decreased activity of the thyroid gland and dexedrine, for a long time the principal ingredient of slimming pills is undesirable as it is a drug of addiction. The fact that there is no alternative to strict dieting was well appreciated by William Banting, the fashionable undertaker of St James's Street, London, who, having reduced his weight by 46 lb in one year was so delighted that in 1863 he wrote a pamphlet entitled *Letter on Corpulence addressed to the Public*. He then distributed 2,500 copies free of charge followed in 1864 by the printing of a further 50,000 which he sold at 6*d.* a copy. The impact of this pamphlet on the public was such that *Punch* had cartoons about him and *Blackwood's Magazine* lampooned him but, at the same time, the English language gained the new word, 'banting', which the *Concise Oxford Dictionary* defines as the 'treatment of obesity by abstinence from sugar, starch and fat'.

Banting described in his pamphlet how, finding in his early thirties that he was becoming overweight, he consulted an eminent surgeon who recommended him to take up rowing. Of this, Banting says, 'It is true I gained muscular vigour but with it a prodigious appetite, which I was compelled to indulge and consequently increased in weight'. After this he consulted many other authorities and on their advice, in addition to rowing, tried sea-bathing, walking and horse-riding: drank enormous quantities of physic and frequented the spas of Leamington, Cheltenham and Harrogate, but all to no avail. The slightest movement was accompanied by much puffing and blowing, he could not stoop to tie his shoes, 'nor attend to the little offices humanity requires without considerable pain and difficulty'. Turkish baths had become fashionable by the middle of the nineteenth century but after a course of ninety of these he had lost not more than 6 lb. His discomfort was such that he had to go downstairs slowly and backwards and at last, finding his sight was failing and his hearing impaired, he consulted, in August 1862, an unnamed but eminent ear specialist. He, according to Banting, 'made light of the case, looked into my ears, sponged them internally and blistered them outside, without the slightest benefit, neither enquiring into any of my bodily ailments which he probably thought unnecessary, nor affording me even time to name them'. It was fortunate for Banting that being August the specialist left town for his

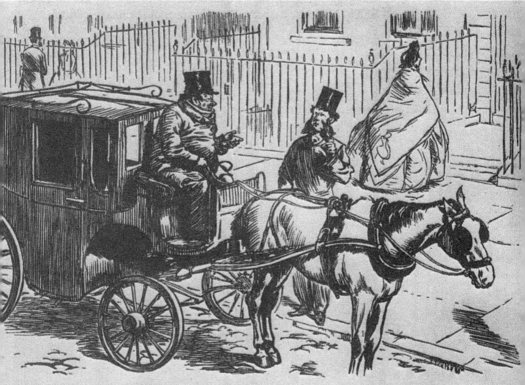

ll (to Corpulent Cabman). "HAW, HERE'S SIXPENCE—GET YOURSELF—GLASS—BEER."
bby. "THANK YOU, SIR, ALL THE SAME; BUT I NEVER TAKE IT. I'M A FOLLERIN' MR. BANTIN'S ADWICE FOR CORPULENCE, SIR.
s, I MAY TAKE TWO OR THREE GLASSES O' GOOD CLARET, OR A GLASS OR TWO OF SHERRY WINE, OR RED PORT, OR MADEIRY;
T O' SPERITS——" *(Swell, deeply touched, makes the Sixpence Half-a-Crown.)*

Cartoon from 'Punch', 1864, showing Cabby following Mr Banting's advice annual holiday because this compelled him to seek other assistance and happily this time he found an ear specialist who not only recognised that all his troubles were due to corpulence but prescribed for him a special diet. This specialist was unnamed in Banting's pamphlet but in 1864, because hundreds of people had written to him asking for this doctor's name he revealed that it was Mr William Harvey, F.R.C.S., of Soho Square, London. 'To name Mr Harvey might appear like a puff which I know he abhors; indeed I should prefer not to do so now...' By the time Banting became his patient, Harvey certainly needed no public recommendation and indeed must have found it distinctly embarrassing for he was a well-established specialist in aural diseases, on the staff of the Great Northern Hospital. It was the publicity he received in connection with Banting's pamphlet that persuaded him to write his book *On Corpulence in relation to Disease, with some remarks on Diet.*

There is no doubt that if more people followed Mr Banting's diet today their general health would improve and their liability to disease and in particular coronary thrombosis would be much reduced.

14

The heart under pressure

IT must always have been common knowledge that on occasions
blood spurts from the body under pressure, but it was Harvey's
observation that this only happens when arteries are severed, in
contrast to the slow manner in which it drips from damaged veins,
that assisted him in his discovery of the circulation of the blood. The
next important step, of measuring this arterial pressure, was not
made until seventy-five years after Harvey's death and then, perhaps
surprisingly, by a churchman, the Reverend Stephen Hales (1677–
1761). Hales was a most interesting and versatile person who, having
graduated as a Bachelor of Arts at Cambridge in 1696 was appointed
a Fellow of Corpus Christi College and it was there, in 1704, the year
after he became a Master of Arts, that he met William Stukeley.
Hales and Stukeley, finding they had much in common, became
close friends and spent many hours together studying natural history,
anatomy and chemistry. They searched for fossils, chased butterflies,
dissected dogs, frogs and other animals, in addition to repeating some
of the classic scientific work already performed by Robert Boyle.
When Hales left Cambridge he became curate at the parish church of
St Mary's, Teddington, Middlesex, where he remained for the rest
of his long life, except for a period each summer when he visited
Farringdon in Hampshire, after his appointment as Rector there. In
addition to being a diligent minister he pursued the study of science
so successfully and made such notable original contributions that in
1718 he was appointed a Fellow of the Royal Society. The enthusiastic reception by the Society and, in particular, by its President
Isaac Newton, of his reports of some classical experiments on the
effects of the sun in causing sap to rise in trees, encouraged him to
continue his studies which culminated in the publication, in 1727,
of a book entitled *Vegetable Staticks*. In this work he described many
quantitative experiments on plant function including the measure-
ment of the force with which sap rises in stems. It was this estimation
of sap pressure that induced him next to measure the pressure of

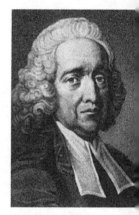

*Rev. Stephen Hales
(1677–1761)*

blood in arteries. He achieved this by inserting a glass tube, the first manometer ever to be used, into horses' arteries so that he could estimate the pressure by measuring the height to which the blood rose in the tube. In his book, *Statical Essays: containing Haemastaticks; or An Account of some Hydraulick and Hydrostatical Experiments made on the Blood and Blood Vessels of Animals*, first published in 1733 he gives details of eleven experiments. In the first experiment he describes how he caused a live mare, about fourteen years of age, to be tied to the ground on her back. He opened the femoral artery and inserted into it a brass pipe attached to which was a vertical glass tube nine feet in length. When the ligature on the artery was untied the blood gradually rose in the tube until eventually it was eight feet three inches above the level of the heart. He admits the procedure caused the horse pain and that because of this her pulse rate was sometimes 60 or 100 a minute in comparison with a horse's normal rate, when not frightened or in pain, of about 36 a minute, and concludes that this factor may have increased the pressure above normal. He then bled the animal and after each quart of blood had escaped, took the pressure again, until finally after about fifteen quarts of blood had been evacuated the mare broke out into cold clammy sweats before she finally died. He found that for the most part the pressure became less with increasing blood loss but that on some occasions, because of violent straining of the mare in an attempt to get loose, the pressure was higher than expected. In his second experiment, a month later, he had an eleven-year-old gelding thirteen hands high, tied to the ground on its back. He fixed the same brass pipe and glass tube to the left femoral artery and repeated the same experiment of measuring the blood pressure after successive bleedings. At one stage he tried to block the horse's nostrils to see the effects on the pressure of laboured respirations and stated that he would have continued the experiment almost to the point of suffocation had the horse not struggled so violently that he had to take the tube out of the artery. In the third experiment he measured the pressure in the left carotid artery of a white mare and this time used the windpipe of a goose to join the brass pipe to the glass tube. He did this because, the windpipe being flexible allowed the animal to move its head without interfering with the readings. Again, repeated blood pressure measurements were taken after successive amounts of blood had been withdrawn, until death ended the experiment. At the end of the third experiment, after the horse had died, he made a cast of the left ventricle by filling it with melted beeswax so that he could estimate the size of the chamber by measuring the amount of fluid displaced when the cast was immersed in water. Finding that this was one hundred and sixty cubic centimetres and knowing that the average pulse rate of a horse is 36 per minute he estimated the cardiac output of a horse at rest to be six litres of blood per minute. From his other measurements in these experiments he concluded that the blood pressure in man would be equal to a column of blood seven and a half feet high. This was a somewhat high estimate but a remarkable approximation considering the limitations of his method. The horses used in his experiments were some which, because they were no longer fit for service, were awaiting slaughter. In the remainder of his experiments similar observations were made on sheep, deer and dogs.

At first sight it may appear strange to find a practising minister engaged in such experiments, but it was not unusual in those days for churchmen to take an active part in science and in his letter, dedicating his book to King George II he said:

the study of nature will ever yield us fresh matter of entertainment, and we have great reason to bless God for the faculties and abilities he has given us, and the strong desire he has implanted in our minds, to search into and contemplate his works, in which the farther we go, the more we see the signatures of his wisdom and power, everything pleases and instructs us because in everything we see a wise design.

His interests embraced many aspects of science as may be judged from the further work published in 1739 and this time dedicated to the Lords of the Admiralty, which he entitled 'Philosophical experiments: containing useful and necessary instructions for such as undertake long Voyages at Sea: showing how Salt-water may be made fresh, wholesome, and how Fresh water may be preserved sweet: how Biscuits, corn, etc. may be secured from the Weevil Maggots and other Insects; and Flesh preserved in Hot Climates by salting Animals whole; to which is added an account of Experiments, and Observations on Chalybeate or Steel-waters, with some Attempts to convey them to distant places, preserving their virtues to a greater degree than has hitherto been done; likewise a proposal for cleansing away Mud, etc. out of Rivers, Harbours and Reservoirs.' Two years later he designed a ventilator for the removal of foul air from the lower decks of ships, a device which, when later fitted to the roof of Newgate Prison, was responsible for a considerable reduction in the death rate there from gaol fever. His scientific inventiveness was also put to good purpose in his parish, so that, with his help, the village obtained a supply of pure water; also he helped to construct the church lantern and replaced the wooden tower which held it by one made of brick.

He died on 4 January 1761 at the age of eighty-four, and in accordance with his wishes his body was placed under the new tower of the church. There is also a monument in Westminster Abbey.

The glass tube used for measuring the pressures in Hales's experiments was inconveniently long and cumbersome. The next practical step was taken by Poiseuille who, in France in 1828, was able to use a much shorter one by filling a U-tube with mercury, the first occasion when the arterial blood pressure was measured, as it is now, in terms of millimetres of mercury. From Hales's observation that the blood from the carotid artery rose to a height of eight to nine feet in the measuring tube whereas that from the jugular vein was less than a foot high, led the rector to assume, and the belief persisted for another century, that the arterial pressure, once the blood leaves the heart, gradually becomes less as it travels along the smaller peripheral arteries towards the veins. Poiseuille, the first man to use an anti-coagulant in his arterial cannulae, was able, by using cannulae of decreasing size, to measure the pressure in all sizes of arteries from the largest to some of the smallest and found that the same pressure is maintained throughout the entire course of the arterial system.

The direct reading of the blood pressure by inserting a cannula into an artery has obvious disadvantages and thus it was a great advance when indirect methods were devised. Karl Vierordt in 1854 attempted to do this in Germany by seeing how many weights had to be added to a scale pan attached to a lever pressed on to the radial artery in order to obliterate the pulse. But the first man to make systematic and important observations of the arterial blood pressure in health and disease was Frederick Akhbar Mahomed (1849–84). His grandfather, an Indian physician in the service of the East India Company, on his retirement settled in Brighton where he opened a shampoo and vapour bath business. This became so fashionable and successful that ultimately he was appointed Shampoo Surgeon to Their Majesties George IV and William IV. Frederick began the study of medicine at Guy's Hospital in 1869. While still a student he became interested in Marey's sphygmograph and modified the instrument so that the pressure on the button overlying the radial artery could be adjusted by a thumbscrew connected to a dial which recorded the force exerted in ounces troy weight. His routine use of this sphygmomanometer in cases of scarlet fever admitted to the London Fever Hospital when he was the Resident Medical Officer there for a short time, enabled him to recognise that a raised blood pressure is an early sign of what is now known as acute nephritis, a disease which, like rheumatic fever, at times complicates streptococcal infections including scarlet fever. There is no doubt that his interest in disorders of the kidney had been stimulated by the important work on the subject by Richard Bright, the Guy's Hospital physician who died eleven years before Mahomed became a medical student. Mahomed was not only the first man to discover that high

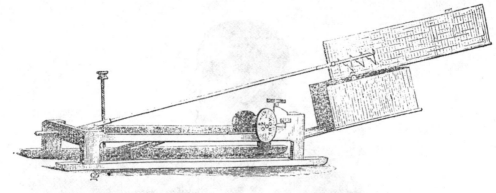

The first sphygmomanometer: Mahomed's modification of a sphygmograph enabling him to measure the blood pressure in ounces troy weight

blood pressure is a feature of acute nephritis but that this may be detected before albumin appears in the urine. His paper on the subject appeared in 1874. A year later he was appointed a medical tutor at St Mary's Hospital, Paddington, but returned to Guy's Hospital as a medical registrar in 1878 and was elected to the senior staff of that hospital as an assistant physician in 1881. He contributed several further papers to the medical literature describing the high blood pressure complicating acute and chronic renal disorders, but in addition presented evidence to show that it most commonly occurred without evidence of any underlying disease in the condition now known as essential hypertension. It is most unfortunate that his work for a long time was overlooked and that he did not receive the credit due to him. It is sad too that his promising career was prematurely ended in 1884 when he died of typhoid fever at the age of thirty-five.

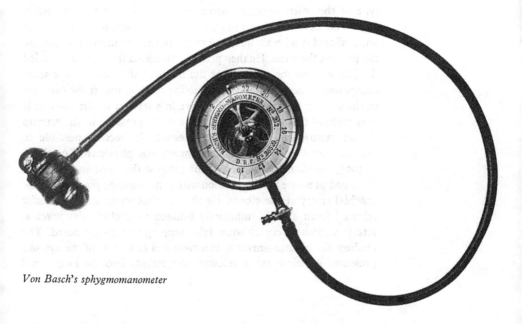

Von Basch's sphygmomanometer

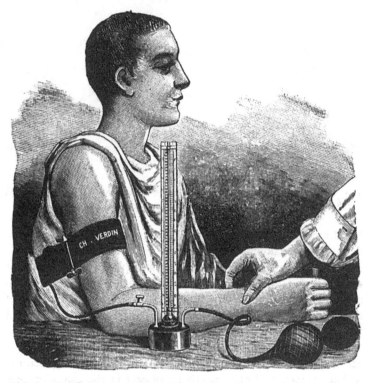

Riva-Rocci's sphygmomanometer

Von Basch, Professor of Medicine in Vienna introduced a much more compact and accurate sphygmomanometer in 1887 which, with a spring plunger to compress the artery at the wrist, recorded the pressure on an aneroid gauge in millimetres of mercury. The prototype of the instrument in current use was devised by the Italian physician, Riva-Rocci in 1896 who, placing a band round the upper arm, inflated it with air until the pressure was sufficient to obliterate the pulse at the wrist. He then gradually released the air and recorded the pressure on the manometer the moment the pulse at the wrist reappeared. This measured the systolic pressure, that is the pressure in the arteries when the ventricles are in a state of contraction. It is now realised that of more significance is the pressure in the arteries during ventricular relaxation or diastole. It became possible to measure both these pressures when the Russian physician, Korotkow, in 1905, abandoned palpation of the pulse at the wrist and recorded the blood pressure by auscultation with a stethoscope placed over the brachial artery at the elbow. He showed that when air is gradually released from a cuff, sufficiently inflated to occlude the brachial artery, a moment comes when faint tapping sounds are heard. The reading on the manometer at this time is a reflection of the systolic pressure. As more air is released the sounds become louder and clearer and then suddenly begin to fade, the reading at this point representing the diastolic pressure.

Since Mahomed's pioneer studies much work has been done in an attempt to identify the diseases associated with elevation of the blood pressure and in trying to explain some of the mechanisms by which this change takes place. At present, in spite of intensive and complex methods of investigation a discoverable underlying cause for a persistently raised blood pressure is found in only about 20 per cent of cases. Most of these is where hypertension is secondary to various types of kidney disease with, in addition, a few cases associated with hormonal disturbances of the adrenal glands or congenital narrowing of the aorta. The great majority of people with a high blood pressure have no detectable underlying disorder of any organ and for this reason are referred to as cases of essential hypertension. The remainder of this chapter, therefore, will be restricted to a discussion of this most common form of high blood pressure.

The average blood pressure for a group of healthy people in early adult life is about one hundred and twenty millimetres of mercury during cardiac systole and eighty millimetres of mercury during diastole. This rises gradually over the years so that at the age of sixty it is usually about one hundred and sixty systolic and ninety diastolic. Any pressure appreciably above the normal for a particular age is called essential hypertension. Although Mahomed first drew attention to this condition it was not well recognised in clinical practice until Sir Clifford Allbutt, in an attempt to distinguish it from high blood pressure secondary to renal disease, referred to it in 1894, as hyperpiesia but the term essential or primary hypertension has now become firmly established.

The cause of essential hypertension is unknown but there is little doubt that heredity plays a part for it is common to find it in more than one member of a family. This was first recognised by Wilhelm Weitz when in 1923 at the Polyklinik at Tübingen he studied eighty-two patients with essential hypertension and compared them with two hundred and fifty-seven patients of similar age attending the clinic for reasons not related to the heart or blood vessels. He found no correlation between high blood pressure and hard physical labour or excessive indulgence in tobacco or alcohol. He was able to relate it to only one factor, namely heredity, as 76·8 per cent of the parents of his patients with hypertension had a history of death from disease of the heart or blood vessels, but only 30·3 per cent of the parents of his controls. He then measured the blood pressure in the siblings of his hypertensive patients as well as in a number of controls of a similar age. He found that for any given age group the percentage of hypertensives among relatives of his patients was greater than in the controls. His studies led him to the view that the disease was inherited as a Mendelian dominant, a conclusion supported by Sir Robert Platt of Manchester, whose study of heredity in hypertension was published in 1947.

In 1954 Professor Pickering and his colleagues published results of a survey in which they studied the blood pressures in a group of first-degree relatives of patients with essential hypertension, a group of first-degree relatives of patients without essential hypertension and a control group from the general population. They found that the pattern of blood pressure readings in the relatives of subjects without hypertension were indistinguishable from those of the control group and that both showed a gradual increase with age: they found that the relatives of subjects with essential hypertension also show a similar rate of rise in blood pressure with age but that for any given age group the pressure is at a higher level. Further, that the greater the deviation of the patient's blood pressure from normal for someone of that age and sex the greater is the deviation of the blood pressure of their first-degree relatives, suggesting that it is not hypertension alone but the degree of hypertension that is inherited. Any harm that may result from a blood pressure raised above the normal for age and sex depends on its severity, the age at which it first appears and the sex of the person. In general women withstand a raised blood pressure better than men but in both sexes an appreciably raised pressure in early adult life is bound to cause trouble. The blood pressure may remain raised for many years without producing any symptoms with the muscle of the left ventricle undergoing compensatory hypertrophy or thickening but after a time the persistent strain results in heart failure. The increased pressure within the blood vessels also leads to thickening of the walls of the medium sized arteries, a change which may be obvious on feeling the pulse at the wrist, but in addition the physician learns much about the state of the arteries by observing the condition of the vessels in the retina at the back of the eye with the aid of an ophthalmoscope. The importance of this examination was first stressed in 1876 by William Gowers when an assistant physician at University College Hospital in London.

This thickening of the walls of the arteries which occurs in hypertension is the result of hypertrophy of the muscle layers and has to be distinguished from the atheromatous deposits on the inside of the walls which cause narrowing of the lumen of these vessels. This degenerative process occurs independently of a raised blood pressure although the latter hastens its progress. It is for this reason that the incidence of coronary artery occlusive disease is higher in hypertensive subjects. The arteries of the brain too are more often narrowed by atheroma in people with a raised blood pressure making them more liable to the development of strokes. Headaches however are not a typical feature of uncomplicated essential hypertension but often occur once a person is told that his blood pressure is high, because of associated anxiety.

The kidneys are not affected and renal failure is not a feature of straightforward essential hypertension but some people develop hypertension secondary to chronic infection of the kidneys and also serious renal changes occur in the accelerated or malignant type of hypertension. This condition, fortunately uncommon, affecting mostly men in early middle age is, as its name implies, very serious and in addition to the development of renal failure, intense spasm of the cerebral vessels leads to the occurrence of severe headaches, fits and at times unconsciousness.

Emotional strain is well known to cause a temporary rise in blood pressure and is often the cause of the transient increase which may occur during the ordeal of a medical examination and for this reason most life insurance companies insist that a raised blood pressure reading has to be checked on more than one occasion. A consistently high pressure carries a decreased expectation of life and therefore in all except the elderly, requires treatment. Low sodium diets, at one time fashionable, are no longer employed but obesity has to be corrected as this also is associated with decreased longevity and because weight reduction is often associated with a fall in blood pressure. The aggravating effect of constant emotional stress often has to be controlled by suitable sedation. In addition however many cases require the use of specific hypotensive drugs.

Since Gaskell and Langley, towards the end of the last century, first elucidated the mechanism of the autonomic nervous system, it has been known that the blood pressure is influenced by the action of parasympathetic and sympathetic nerves on the heart and blood vessels, also that this action may be affected by changes taking place in the autonomic control centres in the brain or at nerve endings or in the ganglia or relay stations situated along the course of these nerves. Langley showed that the transmission of impulses across ganglia may be effected by drugs when in 1889 he demonstrated that nicotine applied to them temporarily improved conduction and then stopped it altogether. Since that time there has been a search amongst synthetic chemical substances in an attempt to find potent ganglion-blocking drugs which would lower the blood pressure. The first such drug to be used at all widely for this purpose was tetraethylammonium but this was supplanted in 1950 by the methonium group of drugs with hexamethonium the first clinically useful one, and others have been introduced since. The ganglion-blocking group of drugs lower the blood pressure by reducing the constrictor effect of the sympathetic nerves on arteries and veins thereby reducing the peripheral vascular resistance and the cardiac output. Unfortunately, in addition they block the parasympathetic ganglia and because of this cause a wide range of unpleasant side effects. Therefore, their use has now been abandoned in favour of drugs whose action is only on the sympathetic system preventing the release of noradrenaline at its nerve ending. Examples of such adrenergic neurone-blocking drugs are guanethidine, which at the present time is extensively used, and the shorter acting bethanidine. Another useful drug is methyl-dopa, a substance which interferes with the synthesis of noradrenaline in the body.

At the same time as advances in hypotensive treatment have been made from studies of synthetic substances in the laboratory, progress has been made by observation of the action of a naturally growing shrub in India. For centuries extracts of a certain plant have been used in primitive Hindu medicine for a variety of conditions including insomnia, insanity and, because of the resemblance of its root to a snake, for snake bite. In 1703 this plant was named *Rauwolfia serpentina* in honour of Dr Leonhard Rauwolf of Algsberg, a six-teenth-century botanist who incidentally had never seen the plant or known of its existence. Its introduction into scientific medicine was in 1931 when Sen and Bose described, in the *Indian Medical Journal*, the ability of this drug to lower a raised blood pressure. Its use however was limited until 1949 when Vakil reported its action in the *British Heart Journal*. Rauwiloid contains many alkaloids including reserpine, currently in use as a hypotensive agent. Its action on the autonomic nervous system has been found to be both central and peripheral.

As all the drugs available for the treatment of high blood pressure are liable to produce side effects they have to be employed under close medical supervision with the dose of certain of them, including guanethidine and methyldopa, carefully adjusted to each individual's requirements. In order to reduce these toxic effects to a minimum it is often better for a small amount of several of them to be given rather than a large amount of any one. Fortunately, when in 1957 the diuretic chlorothiazide, the action of which will be discussed in the chapter on heart failure, was discovered, it was soon found to have the additional important action of potentiating the effect of hypotensive drugs; therefore, it is often prescribed in combination with them so that their dose may be reduced.

The introduction of powerful hypotensive drugs during the last twenty years has been a major advance enabling dangerous levels of high blood pressure to be brought under good control. The search however still continues for other drugs, the specific hypotensive effect of which is not complicated by other undesirable actions.

15

Invasion of the heart by bacteria

DAMAGE to the valves and heart muscle in rheumatic fever, the most common acquired disease of the heart, does not occur because of direct bacterial invasion but arises from a hypersensitivity reaction to bacteria elsewhere in the body. Bacterial endocarditis on the other hand, as its name implies, is a condition where the tissues of the heart are directly attacked by bacteria circulating in the blood. It does not however affect a normal heart but only one already damaged by rheumatic fever or malformed from some congenital defect.

Sir William Osler, who was the first to recognise the disease, described it in 1885 as an acute fulminating condition but later, in 1908, showed that more commonly it followed a more chronic insidious course. Osler (1849–1919), whose observations on angina pectoris have already been discussed, was an exceptional person whose professional life greatly enriched the practice of medicine both in North America and Britain.

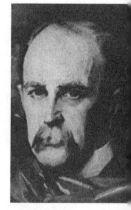

Sir William Osler (1849–1919)

Osler's early life was spent at Bonds Head, Ontario, his father, who was a Canon in the Church of England, having emigrated to Canada soon after his marriage. William was a boy of great vitality whose high spirits caused him to be expelled from the local grammar school: it was, however, the liveliness of his personality which led him to excel both in work and athletics in his later school life. His medical training started in 1868 at Toronto and was completed at McGill University where he graduated in 1872. After postgraduate study in London, Berlin and Vienna, he held teaching appointments at McGill, in addition to becoming, when still relatively young, a full physician at the General Hospital, Montreal. In 1884 he moved to the United States, first to the University of Pennsylvania at Philadelphia and later as Physician in Chief at the Johns Hopkins Hospital at Baltimore. His practice of medicine in Canada and America coincided with important developments in the science of bacteriology and his textbook, *The Principles and Practise of Medicine*, published in 1892, was the first comprehensive work to incorporate these advances. It was in Montreal in the early part of his career, when he was working partly in the wards and partly in the Pathology Laboratory that he first came to recognise the symptoms, signs and appearances of the heart in the disease now known as bacterial endocarditis. In Philadelphia several patients with this disease came under his care and it was a study of these which formed the basis of his Goulstonian Lectures which he delivered to the Royal College of Physicians of London in 1885.

Osler was a frequent visitor to England where he felt that he really belonged and hoped that the chance might come for him to settle there. It was therefore with much enthusiasm that he accepted the post of Professor of Medicine at Oxford when this was offered to him in August 1904. His election as a Fellow of the Royal Society, an honour he greatly cherished, had been conferred on him six years previously at a time when Lord Lister was President.

His days at Oxford were supremely happy, marred only by the death of his elder son Edward as a result of wounds received at Ypres in 1917, his younger son having died when a baby. He never fully recovered from the shock of Edward's death and died himself from pneumonia in December 1919.

His contemporaries placed him among the great physicians of all ages. Sir George Newman, at the time of Osler's death said, 'I have a sacred grove for my medical heroes, a sort of spiritual Valhalla, and there you will find Pasteur, Lister, Paget, Hutchinson, and there must now go the youthful-hearted, gay and charming Osler'.

It was while he was at Oxford that in June 1908 he read before the Association of Physicians of Great Britain and Ireland his classic account of 'chronic infectious endocarditis'. He recalled in this paper how he had described, in 1885, a more acute type of infection which kills the patient within several weeks, but said he had come to realise that it was far more common for the disease to take an insidious and protracted course, the fatal termination of which may often be delayed for anything up to a year. He stressed that the infection attacks valves which have already been damaged in the past and described the large, firm, greyish-yellow vegetations which develop on and around the cusps of these valves. These vegetations, when examined under the microscope, are found to consist of masses of fibrin, bacteria and platelets.* As they are extremely friable small fragments are liable to break off and form emboli† which travel in the blood until they

*Platelets—cells normally found in blood where they assist with the mechanism of clotting.
†Embolus—from the Greek for plug or stopper—a clot or other substance carried by the blood from one site to another and forced into a small vessel where it obstructs the circulation.

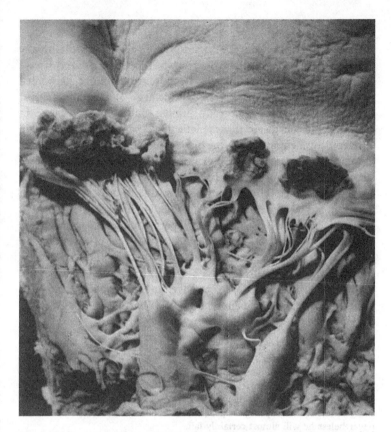

Heart with bacterial endocarditis affecting the mitral valve and showing typical large friable vegetations (in contrast to the small bead-like vegetations which appear on the valves in rheumatic fever (see illustration on page 45)

become plugged in the small terminal vessels of distant organs. Osler described the damage this may cause to the kidneys, with the appearance of blood in the urine; to the brain with the development of 'strokes', to the eye, with the production of sudden blindness; and to the spleen, with the development of pain; in addition he described the characteristic transient painful erythematous nodules which arise in the skin, also thought to be embolic in origin, which are seen, particularly at the tips of the fingers, and now known as Osler's nodes. Osler said of these nodes:

My attention was first called to these in the patient of Dr Mullen of Hamilton whose description is admirable: 'the spots came out at intervals as small swollen areas, some the size of a pea, others a centimetre and a half in diameter, raised, red, with a whitish point in the centre. I have known them to pass away in a few hours but more commonly they last for a day, or even longer. The commonest situation is near the tip of the finger, which may be slightly swollen.'

Osler made it clear that the diagnosis may be very difficult initially as for weeks, or even months, there may be no evidence of the disease other than persistent fever but that its presence should be considered in any patient with long-standing valve damage who becomes febrile, particularly if murmurs already present undergo any change in character. He considered that the infection is caused by a weak strain of streptococci circulating in the blood and that the clinical diagnosis should always be confirmed by culturing the patient's blood in the laboratory. Subsequent work has confirmed this view and for many years by far the commonest organism was *Streptococcus viridans*, an organism of low virulence commonly found in infected tooth sockets. It was in 1935 that Okell and Elliott reported in the *Lancet* that when teeth are extracted from infected gums 75 per cent of cases develop infection of the blood stream. This septicaemia in otherwise healthy people is transient and harmless but in the presence of heart valve damage from rheumatic fever or congenital malformation leads to a condition which Hadfield and Garrod of St Bartholomew's Hospital, London, said:

presents a paradox for which there is no equivalent, that of a micro-organism of very low pathogenicity causing a disease which is almost invariably fatal, and this in spite of the development of a high degree of humoral resistance. The physician can rarely feel more desperately hopeless than at the bedside of some of these cases, knowing that he has probably months in which to try every means of interrupting the progress of this inexorable infection and that nevertheless he will almost certainly fail.

These words were written in 1942, only a short time before it was discovered that *Streptococcus viridans* infection of the heart valves may be brought under control by the use of penicillin in very large amounts, far exceeding the usual dose required for most infections. The mortality however remained grave in spite of this because cure of the infection was all too often followed by death from heart failure resulting from the extensive damage inflicted on the valves by the infection. In the last ten years cardiac surgeons have been able to improve the outlook considerably by their skilful repair of such valves. Unfortunately, in spite of these advances and the prevention of bacterial endocarditis by giving a short course of penicillin to all patients with valve damage when they have to undergo dental extractions, the downward trend in the mortality of this disease which started when penicillin was discovered has not been sustained during the past decade. In Britain, as the result of treatment with penicillin, the death rate fell from about a thousand cases a year, but since 1954 it has remained fairly constant at about three hundred and fifty a year. The inability to reduce the mortality any further appears to be because the disease has changed its pattern. Formerly it was a disease mainly of younger people but now it is increasingly being seen in those over the age of sixty. The Registrar-General's records show that in 1931 13 per cent of those dying from bacterial endocarditis were over sixty, in 1954 it was 30 per cent and by 1963 it was 47 per cent. Also, although *Streptococcus viridans* may still be the commonest single cause of the condition, infection with other more virulent and often antibiotic-resistant organisms such as the *Streptococcus faecalis* and *Staphylococcus aureus* occur more frequently in older patients. The bacteraemia when it arises in the elderly, does not occur so much from dental extractions as from infections of the urinary tract, gall-bladder and colon. The failure to control some of these infections by penicillin alone and the need so often now to employ various combinations of antibiotics, is an excellent example of the constant battle being waged between man and bacteria.

16

Pump failure

HEART failure occurs when the cardiac muscle, ceasing to be efficient as a pump, is no longer able to maintain an adequate circulation of blood round the body. This may be an acute event such as occurs with a coronary thrombosis when the blood supply to the muscle is suddenly cut off, or a chronic process due to the muscle becoming exhausted from working at a disadvantage for a long period, for example, when a ventricle has to pump blood against the resistance of a high arterial pressure, or when its work is increased because of the faulty action of one or more valves.

Heart failure may affect the right side of the heart, the left side or both. Richard Lower, in his *Tractatus de corde* in 1669, was one of the first to show a grasp of the effects on the circulation of heart failure when he said, 'but when the parenchyma of the heart has been harmed by various diseases ... so that it cannot vibrate or contract without great trouble or difficulty, it soon gives up its motion; whence the movement of the blood also to the same degree becomes weak and languid'. As a result of this slowing of the circulation, blood accumulates in the veins so that the pressure in them rises as may readily be observed in right ventricular failure by examination of the jugular veins in the neck. Normally they cannot be seen but once the right ventricle is unable to perform its function efficiently because of this rise in pressure in the superior vena cava and in the veins returning the blood from the head and neck, the distended walls of the jugular veins become clearly visible. A similar high pressure develops in the inferior vena cava and the veins draining into it from the lower part of the body. As this raised venous pressure causes the various organs in the body to become congested with blood, failure of the right side of the heart is often referred to as congestive cardiac failure. It is this raised venous pressure which forces the fluid part of the blood out of the veins into the surrounding tissues causing them to swell with oedema, the condition formerly known as dropsy. This swelling becomes particularly noticeable in the lower legs and feet especially after prolonged standing.

A similar raised pressure in the pulmonary veins as a result of left ventricular failure causes fluid to exude into the alveoli of the lungs which interferes with the diffusion of oxygen from the air into the blood. This outpouring of fluid into the alveoli in left ventricular failure is frequently sudden and gives rise to severe and terrifying bouts of shortness of breath, often at night when the patient lies down. As such an attack is accompanied by wheezing it may easily be confused with the disease occurring in allergic people known as bronchial asthma and, in fact, a distinction was not made between the two until the early part of the nineteenth century when James Hope referred to the paroxysmal attacks of nocturnal wheezing caused by acute left ventricular failure as cardiac asthma. His description in his book published in 1831 of a patient with this condition is remarkably vivid:

... with eyes widely expanded and starting, eyebrows raised, nostrils dilated, a ghastly and haggard countenance, and the head thrown back at every inspiration, he casts round a hurried, distracted look of horror, of anguish, and of supplication; now imploring, in plaintive moans, or quick, broken accents, and half-stifled voice, the assistance already often lavished in vain; now upbraiding the impotency of medicine; and now, in an agony of despair, drooping his head on his chest and muttering a fervent invocation for death to put a period to his sufferings. For a few hours—perhaps only for a few minutes—he tastes an interval of delicious respite which cheers him with the hope that the worst is over, and that his recovery is at hand. Soon that hope vanishes. From a slumber fraught with the horrors of a hideous dream, he starts up with a wild exclamation that 'It is returning'. At length after reiterated recurrences of the same attacks, the muscles of respiration, subdued by efforts of which the instinct of self-preservation alone renders them capable, participate in the general exhaustion and refuse to perform their function. The patient gasps, sinks, and expires.

When a raised arterial pressure or faulty action of a damaged valve, throws an increased load on one of the ventricles, it does not immediately go into failure but undergoes elongation and enlargement of its muscle fibres in order to increase its power of contraction sufficiently to maintain an efficient circulation for many years. The thickening, or hypertrophy, of the muscle results in a marked enlargement of the affected chamber and its increased force of action is often apparent to the patient as well as observable by the physician. As this enlargement is compensatory no measures should be taken to reduce it but unfortunately this was not appreciated by the earlier physicians. Corvisart, thinking that the enlargement and the associated increased activity of the heart was harmful attempted to weaken its action by general measures designed to diminish the strength of the patient, and because of this he and his pupil Laënnec recommended that patients should be starved and repeatedly bled. It was for the same reason that the French physician, René Bertin, in 1824, in writing about the treatment of heart disease, said that the measures to be employed against hypertrophy should be 'essentially antiphlogistic' and calculated to produce debility. This attitude towards treatment, however, was before long to have its critics, one of the foremost being Sir Dominic Corrigan, the Irish physician. From his paper, 'On Permanent Patency of the Mouth of the Aorta', published in 1832, it is clear that he appreciated the value of hypertrophy for he asked the pertinent question, 'Is this hypertrophy disease, or is it a wise provision of nature by which the organ is thus made equal to the increased labour it has to perform?' His answer was clear and uncompromising, 'It is at once obvious that to interfere with this wise provision of nature, to diminish the strength of the heart, or if we choose other words, to direct, according to the advice of Laënnec, Bertin, etc. our measures against the hypertrophy of the organ, is to deprive the system of the only power which enables the heart to carry on the circulation.' He therefore recommended that instead of measures designed to weaken the patient on the contrary the general constitution should be strengthened by a generous diet but with at the same time abstinence from beverages such as malt liquors. That, in addition, cardiac patients should be encouraged to live as normally as possible and not indiscriminately be prohibited from work regardless of the individual circumstances.

Among the many cases which led him to adopt this enlightened view was that of a young man who, when found to have heart disease, was in a good general state of health but, to quote Corrigan, 'bleeding after bleeding, and blister after blister, were repeated, starvation enforced and digitalis exhibited, until the patient was reduced to such weakness that he had scarcely strength to raise himself in bed'. The treatment was only stopped when the patient's death appeared imminent. From that moment the man improved and several years later Corrigan was able to report, 'the patient is still alive, the disease is still present; but, with full living and good air, he is able not only to take considerable exercise, but even to undertake the fatigue of a business that constantly requires very laborious exertion'.

Physicians therefore had to decide not only the proper indications for treatment but also as to what measures were most appropriate. William Withering had already given an excellent guide when he pointed out the remarkable improvement he had observed in patients whose dropsy was dispersed by an increased flow of urine from the action of digitalis. He not unreasonably thought that digitalis achieved this by acting on the kidneys and it was not until 1799 that John Ferriar first ascribed to digitalis a primary action on the heart with the diuretic effect secondary to this and occurring as a result of the improved circulation to the kidneys. Withering was very conscious of the fact that in order to gain the optimum benefit from digitalis it must be employed skilfully, to avoid the poisonous effects of over-dosage. Physicians for the most part of the nineteenth century never learned how to administer it properly. At the time when measures designed to weaken the patient were thought to assist in controlling the overactivity of a damaged heart digitalis was given in sufficient quantity to produce vomiting and diarrhoea. Corrigan, in spite of his enlightened views on the management of heart disease, could have had no idea how to prescribe digitalis because he considered that it had a weakening effect on the heart and aggravated the patients' sufferings; also that often patients only recovered when digitalis was omitted and they were put on stimulants. The indications for use of the drug and its dosage continued to be ill defined until towards the end of the nineteenth century when Mackenzie drew attention to its remarkable effect in the control of the dangerous form of arrhythmia known as auricular fibrillation where the auricles, in a state of ineffectual writhing, cause the ventricles to beat very rapidly and irregularly, both in the timing and force of their contractions. Digitalis, by its specific action on the conduction tissue, blocks many of the impulses from the auricles so that the ventricles, while still remaining irregular in action can be made to beat more efficiently at a rate of about 80 a minute. It is now usual to employ digoxin which is a pure glycoside derivative of digitalis but Mackenzie used a tincture, the strength of which was difficult to standardise. This led him to adopt a method whereby he gave enough of the drug to pro-duce the symptoms of overdosage and from this calculated the optimum amount required for each individual patient. It is clear, from the third edition of his book on diseases of the heart, published in 1914, that he was well aware that there is a danger of sudden and unexpected death when excessive amounts of the drug are prescribed for too long a period, a risk which was not sufficiently appreciated by doctors in general at that time. The teaching of Mackenzie and his pupil, Thomas Lewis, about this drug, and their demonstration of its remarkable efficiency in the management of auricular fibrillation, led to its almost exclusive use for this purpose until well into the twentieth century. It has only been during comparatively recent years that its effect on the failing but regularly beating heart muscle has again been adequately recognised. The present views on the action of digitalis were admirably discussed in the 1963 William Withering Lecture by Sir John McMichael, Director of Medicine at the British Postgraduate Medical School, whose research into the action of this drug, in conjunction with E. P. Sharpey-Schafer in the years immediately after the Second World War was so useful. Now it is realised that by stimulation of the vagus nerve it slows the heart;

by a direct action on the cardiac muscle when in failure it increases its power of contraction; by its effect on the conduction tissue linking the auricles and ventricles it reduces the ventricular rate when the auricles are fibrillating; and finally, by its beneficial effect on a disordered heart it improves the circulation in general, including that to the kidneys, so that by promoting an increased excretion of urine it rids the body of excess fluid accumulated in the tissues.

Although it was the diuretic effect of digitalis which so impressed Withering, more powerful drugs for this purpose have since been discovered. Inorganic mercury salts had been used both as diuretics and for their beneficial action against syphilis for about the last three hundred years. When advances in chemistry led to the synthesis of organic compounds of mercury, one of them, merbaphen, was tried on syphilitic patients undergoing treatment in a Viennese hospital in 1919. It was quickly noticed that although the drug's effect on syphilis was limited it had a pronounced diuretic action. It was for this reason next given to patients in heart failure with considerable benefit. As however certain toxic effects restricted its use, other organic mercury preparations were tested with mersalyl, a combination of mercury and theophylline, remaining the diuretic of choice for the treatment of cardiac failure until ten years ago. One of its disadvantages is that it has to be given by intramuscular injection and mainly for this reason has been supplanted in recent years by other drugs given by mouth. The discovery of these oral diuretics was a chance finding linked with the development of the antibacterial drugs, the sulphonamides, over thirty years ago, about the same time as an enzyme, carbonic anhydrase, was found in red cells which catalyses the reaction in the body between carbon dioxide and water with the formation of carbonic acid. It was observed that sulphanilamide, the first of the sulphonamides, by inhibiting the action of this enzyme, acted as a weak diuretic. This led to the synthesis of other substances of similar chemical composition in the hope that one might be found, the anti-enzymic activity of which is more powerful. This culminated in the discovery of acetazolamide, a potent carbonic anhydrase inhibitor, but a drug whose diuretic effect was found to be disappointing. The search therefore continued and as a result certain benzenedisulphonamides were examined which, paradoxically, although not acting against the enzyme, were nevertheless found to be powerful diuretics. The first to be synthesized by Novello and Sprague in 1957 was chlorothiazide and since then many others have been introduced, some of the more recent ones, including frusemide, triamterene and ethacrynic acid, being so powerful that they have to be administered with great care in order to avoid dangerous dehydration.

17

Congenital heart disease

CONGENITAL heart disease occurs in approximately 0·3 per cent of all live births. Some abnormalities arise because of arrest of embryological development at an early stage, with failure of the primitive sac to divide into four separate chambers. Others are due to faults in the development of the valves. The cause of these errors is for the most part unknown, although oxygen deprivation of the foetus, infection, immunological disturbance, vitamin deficiencies, in addition to genetic abnormalities, have all been postulated. There is, however, a clear relationship between maternal rubella (German measles) acquired in the first four months of pregnancy and developmental defects in the foetus including cataract, glaucoma, deaf mutism, in addition to developmental disorders of the heart. Although foetal injury is not inevitable and a proportion of women who contract rubella in early pregnancy have normal babies, it is obviously better for them to have had the disease before reaching the age of child-bearing and there is therefore much to be said for purposely exposing schoolgirls to the infection rather than protecting them from it. The number of cases of congenital heart disease secondary to rubella is probably less than 2 per cent and in most cases of cardiac malformation there is no obvious environmental cause. Also, the large majority of babies with such defects come from families without other evidence of hereditary congenital malformation. There are a small number of well-documented cases of families in which the same type of developmental error of the heart has occurred in two or three successive generations but these are exceptions. The birth of a child with a structural fault in the heart should not deter a mother from having further children since the risk that subsequent siblings will have similar trouble is extremely small. There is, none the less, good evidence that factors concerned with congenital malformations can be genetically transferred as may be seen from studying families with hereditary disorders of connective tissue such as arachnodactyly and gargoylism, both of which may be associated with developmental

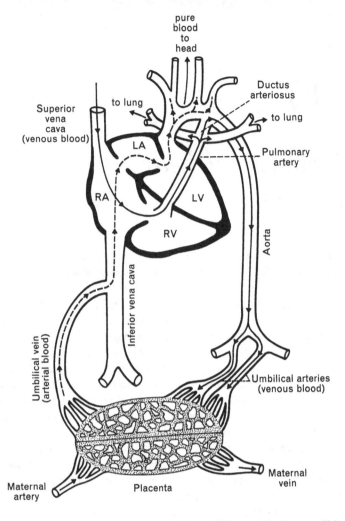

pure
blood
to
head

Ductus
arteriosus

to lung

Superior
vena
cava
(venous blood)

to lung

LA

Pulmonary
artery

RA

LV

RV

Aorta

Inferior vena cava

Umbilical vein
(arterial blood)

Umbilical arteries
(venous blood)

Maternal
vein

The foetal circulation

Maternal
artery

Placenta

errors in the heart. Also from examining children with abnormalities
of the chromosomes such as the mentally defective group known as
mongols, 20 per cent of which have congenital heart disease.

The valves most commonly affected by congenital malformation
are those at the mouth of the pulmonary artery and the mouth of the
aorta. The aortic valve usually has three cusps but sometimes due to
maldevelopment two of them fuse together. This type of bicuspid
valve is particularly prone to a serious form of bacterial infection and
over the years is subject to atheromatous degeneration with the
production of aortic valve stenosis. Children may, somewhat rarely,
be born with a stenosed aortic valve, but far more common is a
congenital stenosis of the pulmonary valve. James Hope gave a good
description in 1839 of the classical murmur and other physical signs
to be found in pulmonary stenosis and contrasted them with those
found in aortic stenosis.

The foetus obtains its oxygen from blood supplied to it from the mother through the veins in the umbilical cord so that during intra-uterine life the lungs remain small and unexpanded with not much blood flowing through them. The oxygenated blood in the umbilical vein flows up the inferior vena cava to reach the right atrium but instead of going from there to the right ventricle and then to the lungs it is diverted into the left atrium through the foramen ovale, a small window in the septum separating the two atria. From the left atrium it passes to the left ventricle for distribution to the body. Blood from the upper part of the body which enters the right atrium from the superior vena cava instead of mixing with the blood from the lower part flows as a separate stream into the right ventricle and then for a short distance up the pulmonary artery before it is diverted through a short channel, the ductus arteriosus, which links the pulmonary artery with the aorta. After birth, when blood has to pass through the lungs for oxygenation, the foramen ovale and ductus arteriosus are sealed off. The foramen ovale remains open in about 10 per cent of the adult population but the hole is usually too small to cause trouble. When however the ductus arteriosus fails to close, because the pressure in the aorta after birth is much higher than in the pulmonary artery, blood now flows in the reverse direction from the aorta to the pulmonary artery so that there is a pathological left to right shunt. This leak of blood from the aorta into the pulmonary circulation increases the work of the left ventricle so that eventually it goes into failure. Another risk, in about a third of all cases, is the development of a serious type of bacterial infection in the walls of the duct.

The existence of the foramen ovale and ductus arteriosus in the foetal circulation has been known for centuries. William Harvey's teacher at Padua, Hieronymus Fabricius, clearly depicted these structures in illustrations, also Harvey gave a good anatomical description of the ductus arteriosus in chapter VI of *De motu cordis*. But the presence of a patent ductus was not diagnosed in life until 1900 when George Gibson, Professor of Medicine in Edinburgh, described the characteristic continuous 'machinery murmur' best heard in the second left intercostal space.

The septa separating the two atria, and the two ventricles, develop by the joining together of tissue growing from more than one point. Failure of fusion results in the persistence of an opening between the two atria (atrial septal defect) or between the two ventricles (ventricular septal defect) allowing oxygenated and deoxygenated blood from the two sides to mix together. The amount of mixing due to 'shunting' of blood from one side to the other obviously depends on the size of the hole. When it is small there may be little or no disturbance

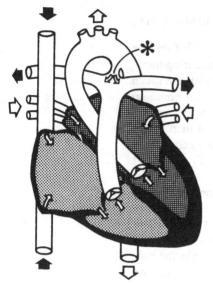

Patent ductus arteriosus

Atrial septal defect. (One type of 'hole in the heart')

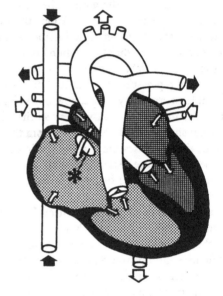

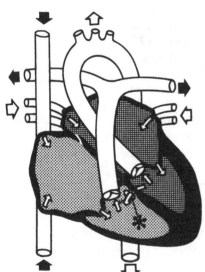

Ventricular septal defect. (Another type of 'hole in the heart')

of the circulation but usually it is large enough to cause varying degrees of disability. These so-called 'holes in the heart' have been much discussed in the Press during recent years since developments in surgical skill have made their repair possible. The most common congenital malformation of the heart is an atrial septal defect. As the pressure of blood in the left atrium after birth is slightly higher than in the right atrium, a septal defect between the two causes part of the oxygenated blood in the left atrium to be shunted into the right atrium with resultant overloading of the right ventricle and pulmonary artery. The size of the defect is variable so that at its worst the entire septum is missing. A person with this type of defect may, therefore, according to the size of the hole, remain symptom free, or develop heart failure in mid-life.

A similar type of defect in the ventricular septum, which is the second most frequent anomaly of the heart, was first described by the French physician Henri Roger in the middle of the last century. Roger who was first in general practice, then later a physician to the hospitals of Paris, was an outstanding clinician whose interest in cardiology and, in particular, the use of the stethoscope in the diagnosis of heart disorders became evident when, in 1839, the Bordeaux Medical and Surgical Society offered a prize for the best paper on the subject, 'To determine what progress has been made in the diagnosis and treatment of diseases, particularly those of the lungs, heart and great vessels, by means of auscultation, either direct or indirect.' Roger, with his colleague Barth, both at that time young house physicians, received an Honourable Mention for their contribution which formed the basis for a more extensive dissertation on auscultation published in 1841. This met with wide acclaim, went through several editions and was translated into many foreign languages. It was in 1879 that Roger presented to the Academy of Medicine his observations on the changes which occur when the septum between the two ventricles remains patent. His attention had first been drawn to the condition many years previously when in his village practice he had heard, in a few of the countless children he examined, a remarkably loud murmur when he placed his stethoscope along the left lower border of the sternum. He pointed out in his paper that this murmur which is accompanied by a purring sensation on placing the hand on the chest, is not only loud but so prolonged that it occupies the entire period of ventricular systole from the first heart sound up to the second heart sound. A murmur with such characteristics would today be called pansystolic and is heard both with ventricular septal defects and when there is incompetence of the mitral valve. Roger correctly taught that a distinction could be made between these two conditions by, amongst other features, a different point of maximum intensity of the murmur. He was surprised to find, when he followed the progress of children with this type of parasternal murmur, that they remained well and free from symptoms for many years. Because of this he felt that the murmur could not be due to any serious inflammation and wondered whether it might possibly be due to some abnormal communication between the two sides of the heart but thought it unlikely however having been taught that this invariably resulted in the mixing of arterial and venous blood with consequent cyanosis of the patient. In 1861 however he was able to prove that this was not always so and to confirm his supposition when, at autopsy examination of a twelve-year-old boy who had died from the complications of a fractured bone, he found that although there had never been any cyanosis during life, there was a large hole in the septum between two ventricles. This congenital malformation had passed unrecognised on the ward, Roger said, due to an 'entirely pardonable omission on a surgical service, the failure to listen to the heart'!

This autopsy discovery rightly convinced him that the distinctive cardiac murmur he had heard in children in the past must have been due to the same type of developmental error. It is now realised that the reason none of the children in his series developed symptoms was because their septal defects were small, a condition known now in his honour as the Maladie de Roger. Larger defects, on the other hand, which allowed shunting of oxygenated blood from the left ventricle to the right ventricle overload the pulmonary circulation and increase the work of the left ventricle with resultant heart failure in middle age or before. At times, because of the increased load on the pulmonary vessels, the pressure in this part of the circulation rises and causes a reverse flow of blood from the right to the left ventricle so that deoxygenated blood passes into the main circulation of the body with consequent cyanosis of the patient.

Roger was also aware that a ventricular septal defect not uncommonly occurs in association with a congenital stenosis of the pulmonary valve. He appreciated that cyanosis must occur with such a combination of disorders as deoxygenated blood not being able to flow freely through the pulmonary artery, is forced through the septal defect into the left ventricle and aorta. It was another Frenchman, Étienne-Louis Arthur Fallot, an eminent teacher in the University of Marseilles who, in 1888, pointed out that the large majority of cases of congenital heart disease in which the patient is cyanosed, the so-called 'blue babies' of modern journalism, have stenosis of the pulmonary artery, a ventricular septal defect, deviation of the origin of the aorta to the right so that blood from both ventricles flows up it, and hypertrophy of the right ventricle. It is because of the combination of these four abnormalities that the condition is often referred to as Fallot's tetralogy. Fallot however was not the first to describe the condition. Credit for this must be given to Niels Stensen who, in the middle of the seventeenth century, gave a clear description of it from his study of an abnormal foetus. He was a remarkable man who in addition to his anatomical studies which included a detailed account of the muscle of the heart, found time to be an expert geologist, physiologist and theologian. It was while on a missionary journey to convert heretics in northern Germany that he died in 1686. It was another hundred years before Sandiford of Leyden in 1777 gave the first account of the physical signs in a child with this disorder. In this country William Hunter, in 1785, also referred to the autopsy findings in two cases: one of which, he said, in life was 'an oppressed miserable looking object' and the other, who lived longer, 'looking like a greyhound ... with legs like a wading waterfowl'. These insensitive phrases might appear to conceal his underlying compassion which led him later in the account to reflect, 'but though the cure of diseases be the first object of our profession, the knowledge of incurable complaints is of much importance to humanity, particularly in restraining us from blistering, vomiting, purging, cutting tissues, applying caustics; in a word, torturing a miserable and incurable human being'. In addition, in 1858, thirty years before Fallot's contribution to the subject, Thomas Peacock gave an excellent account of the tetralogy in an outstanding

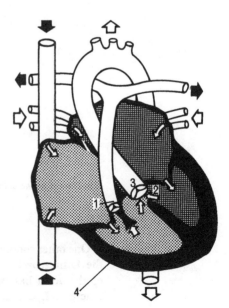

Fallot's tetralogy—commonest cause of 'blue babies'. The four defects can be seen as:
(1) *Narrowing of the mouth of the pulmonary artery (pulmonary stenosis).*
(2) *Defect in the septum separating the two ventricles.*
(3) *Displacement of aorta allowing blood to enter from both ventricles.*
(4) *Hypertrophy or thickening of the wall of the right ventricle*

monograph containing descriptions of various developmental anomalies augmented by superb illustrations.

A striking feature in children suffering from congenital heart disease with cyanosis is the unusual shape of their fingers and in particular of their nails, an appearance commonly known as clubbing of the fingers. One of the early descriptions of this was by Nasse, who described, in 1811, 'nails thicker and more curved, and bent at the front ends over the fingers'. Three years later Farre, in the first comprehensive monograph on congenital defects, referred to a twenty-year-old lad whose fingers, he said, were clubbed at the extremities. This is probably the first time that the term was used. Physicians for a long time considered that such changes were only found in this type of congenital heart disease. In 1824 Elie Gurtrac, of Bordeaux, made it clear that in addition it was present to a lesser degree in patients suffering from pulmonary tuberculosis. His description was excellent, 'the fingers presented at their ends a remarkable swelling; the part supported by the last joint was strikingly enlarged and ended at once in a sort of head and supported a curved nail, wider than it was long'. Since then it has become widely recognised that clubbing of the fingers also occurs in patients with bacterial infection of the heart valves, as well as other lung diseases.

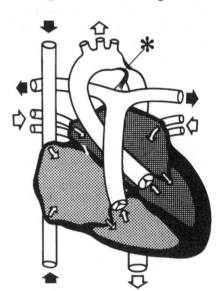

Coarctation of the aorta

One other condition of importance is coarctation of the aorta, from the Latin *coarcto*—to compress, where a short segment of the arch of the aorta has its walls compressed together to form a narrow stricture. Laënnec, in describing a case, said he found the aorta 'contracted to the size of a swan's or even a goose's quill'. It is of particular interest because, as the obstruction to the flow of blood in the aorta occurs beyond the point of origin of the arteries to the head and arms, most of the blood flows into them and only a small quantity trickles past the obstruction to the remainder of the body; therefore, the blood pressure is lower than normal in the lower limbs but abnormally high in the upper limbs so that the condition always has to be considered in a child or young adult found to have a raised blood pressure. The finding of this curious defect at autopsy was remarked upon by Morgagni in 1750 in his eighteenth letter. Now it is possible to demonstrate it in life by taking X-rays after the injection of radio-opaque dyes.

A condition of much interest, but not causing any disability, is dextrocardia where the heart is rotated through 180 degrees so as to lie, for the most part, to the right of the chest. This may lead to temporary confusion on medical examination but nothing worse except when, associated with transposition of the abdominal organs, the condition may lead to serious errors such as the misdiagnosis of an acute appendicitis presenting with pain on the left side. It was the finding of organs reversed in this manner in a soldier in 1686 that led von Leibnitz, the philosopher and writer, to compose the following poem:

> La nature peu sage, et sans doute en debauche
> Placa le foi au côté gauche,
> Et de même, vice versa
> Le cœur à la droite placa.

An English version of which was given by Terence East in his Fitzpatrick Lectures to the Royal College of Physicians in 1956, as follows:

> Nature, unwise and doubtless drunk
> Placed the liver to the left of the trunk
> And likewise, by the same oversight
> Placed the heart across to the right.

Finally, no account of heart disease would be complete without reference to the work of Maude Abbott, of Montreal, who, when in 1899 she was appointed Curator of the McGill University Medical Museum, began a special study of the subject. Her interest, which started when she had to make enquiries about an unlabelled specimen, led eventually to her having an international reputation with material sent to her from all over the world for exact identification. By this means over the years she not only amassed an enormous collection of abnormal hearts but was enabled, in 1936, to publish an analysis of a thousand cases in her *Atlas of Congenital Cardiac Disease*. Her work led to a complete understanding of all the various possible types of congenital cardiac disorders but in spite of this their clinical diagnosis, particularly when more than one anomaly is present at a time, often proves difficult. For a long time this did not matter as the general management was similar for all cases. The spectacular progress in surgery since the Second World War, which has enabled so many different types of malformation to be corrected, has made accurate preoperative diagnosis essential. Fortunately, the concurrent development of complex ancillary diagnostic techniques has been of considerable assistance in this task.

18

The triumphs of surgery

GENERAL interest in the practical possibility of cardiac surgery first
began when Sir Lauder Brunton, consulting physician to St
Bartholomew's Hospital, London, in a short provocative communication to the *Lancet* on 8 February 1902 reflected on the distressing
symptoms of mitral stenosis, and suggested that the protracted
invalidism often associated with this disability warranted the risk of
an operation designed to dilate the narrowed valve orifice. Realising,
he said, that before attempting this in man a suitable technique had
to be evolved from animal experiments, he had obtained the necessary certificates and licence for such work the previous year, but had
only had time to carry out limited experiments on the hearts of
healthy cats as well as practising various methods of dividing stenosed
valves found in diseased hearts at the post-mortem table. He
explained that it was because he had so many other demands on his
time that he had decided to publish a preliminary note in order to
stimulate the interest of others especially surgeons whose final
responsibility it must be to devise the necessary operation. The
response to this was immediate and derogatory. The next week a
leading article in the same journal castigated Sir Lauder for suggesting that others should carry out such a highly dangerous procedure
which he himself had only considered in theory. It discussed the
many risks involved and concluded that there was no evidence that a
valve divided and its aperture enlarged as he had suggested, would
not promptly contract to its former size or worse, or alternatively
that if it did remain open the reflux through it might not be just as
serious. A week later the *Lancet* published a letter from Sir Arbuthnot
Lane, one of the leading surgeons of that time, pointing out that his
colleague Dr Lauriston Shaw had some years before suggested to
him the possibility of operating on mitral stenosis and since then they
had been looking for a suitable patient. Dr Shaw, who later became
a physician at Guy's Hospital, joined in the attack by writing an
irate letter the following week confirming that he had thought of the

operation at least twelve years previously but that he now did not consider it justifiable, adding, 'your readers will I think agree with me that Sir Lauder Brunton's chief task is not to show his surgical colleagues that it is possible to enlarge the stenosed mitral orifice, but to persuade his medical colleagues that such a proceeding is useful. It is possible to do many things that are useless and some things that are harmful.'

The general climate of opinion being against Sir Lauder the matter was not again publicly discussed for some time. He himself, some years later, said that he had intended continuing his experiments but the development of blood poisoning had prevented this. Others however practised the technique in dogs and in 1923 the *Boston Medical and Surgical Journal* published a report by Cutler and Levine giving details of the first patient to be submitted to the operation. This was an eleven-year-old girl with severe narrowing of the mitral orifice which Cutler enlarged by cutting into the cusps with a valvotome, an instrument similar to a slightly curved tonsil knife which he inserted through the left ventricular wall. The patient recovered from the operation and lived for four and a half years but with little improvement in her general condition. Two years later Pribram in Germany also operated on a patient with mitral stenosis using Cutler's technique but the patient died on the sixth post-operative day. In the same year, on 6 May 1925, Henry Souttar, Director of Surgery at the London Hospital, operated on a nineteen-year-old patient. He intended to divide the valve cusps with a knife but before attempting this explored the valve with a finger passed through the left auricular appendage. This revealed to him that although the valve was grossly damaged and incompetent there was only minimal stenosis. It was decided therefore not to carry out valve section as this might increase the degree of reflux but to limit intervention to widening the orifice with the finger. This had little effect on the course of the disease which was most unfortunate as it hindered the development of an operation which was well conceived as shown many years later when dilatation of the mitral valve with a finger inserted into the left atrium in suitably selected cases, proved to be highly successful. Neither Souttar nor any other surgeon attempted the operation again in the immediate future. This might seem surprising but the physicians would not refer any more cases to them principally because Sir James Mackenzie, the foremost cardiologist in those days, was against the procedure and his influence was widespread and powerful. He believed that it was the heart muscle which bore the brunt of the damage in rheumatic fever and that stenosis of the valve was of secondary importance. Sir James even influenced American physicians, except Samuel Levine, in Boston, who encouraged Cutler to operate on six further patients with his valvotome. The results however being disappointing, the operation temporarily fell into disrepute and little further progress in heart surgery was made apart from the repair of certain injuries and various attempts to strip the heart of a thickened pericardium, until the beginning of the Second World War. The impetus which led to a revival in operations on the heart was the development of techniques enabling control of respiration to be maintained once the chest had been opened. Credit for this advance must go to the anaesthetists and in particular to Ivan Magill, consultant anaesthetist to the Westminster and Brompton Hospitals, London, who pioneered much of this work in the years immediately preceding the war. First, it enabled surgeons to remove part or at times the whole of a lung, destroyed by infection or invaded by growth, with relative safety and confidence, while at the same time it gave them the opportunity to get used to working around the heart.

The first outstanding achievement in cardiac surgery was in 1939 when Robert Gross of Boston successfully ligated a patent ductus arteriosus. The operation had originally been suggested in 1907 by John Munro in Boston who practised it on cadavers, not long after Gibson in Edinburgh had described the characteristic machinery noise of this congenital anomaly. But practical application of his idea had to be deferred for at least another thirty years until the complex techniques associated with intrathoracic surgery had been sufficiently developed. The first step was taken by John Strieder who, in 1937, encouraged by the physician Ashton Graybiel of the Massachusetts Memorial Hospital, attempted the operation on a patient with a patent ductus complicated by severe bacterial endocarditis. Although the ductus was successfully ligated, the patient died four days later and when Strieder presented a preliminary report of his operation to the American Association of Thoracic Surgery three months later, no one was sufficiently interested even to comment on it. Robert Gross's successful operation took place fifteen months later. It is interesting that although both worked in Boston, when Gross carried out his operation he was unaware of Strieder's attempt, not having been at the meeting of thoracic surgeons and not at that time knowing Strieder personally. Gross's interest in the work had been stimulated by John Hubbard who was in charge of the Congenital Heart Clinic at the Children's Hospital and before attempting the operation on a patient he worked on animals at the Harvard Medical Laboratory. His success therefore was due partly to careful preparatory work, and also to the fact that they had chosen for their first operation a child who had no complicating infection of the duct or heart. The news of the operation quickly spread throughout the world and other surgeons were encouraged to develop the technique. Maude Abbott, the greatest authority on congenital heart disease, had always con-tended that operating on a patent ductus would be dangerous as it would precipitate the onset of endocarditis. Gross's success dis-proved this belief and in 1943 Touroff, in New York, confirmed Strieder's view that on the contrary the operation would help to combat co-existing infection when he closed the ductus in a patient with a *Streptococcus viridans* endocarditis and all evidence of the infection disappeared. One year later Oswald Tubbs of St Bartholo-mew's Hospital, London, also courageously operated on a patient with a patent ductus arteriosus in the presence of infection with *Haemo-philus influenzae* which as a result of a successful operation was eventually brought under control. These results were particularly impressive as no really effective antibiotics against these organisms were available at that time.

About the same time as this operation was being developed Alfred Blalock who was Professor of Surgery at Vanderbilt University from 1938 to 1941 before holding a similar appointment at Johns Hopkins University, started to develop the technique of linking together or anastomosing major vessels in order to circumvent obstruction to the outflow of blood from the heart. Whilst at Vander-bilt, Blalock, working with S. E. Levy, conducted experiments on dogs in which they anastomosed the left subclavian to the left pulmonary artery. They observed that the dogs, followed for several months, developed no ill effects from this. Later, at Johns Hopkins Hospital, Blalock continued his experiments on dogs and by-passed a gap in the aorta created by operation by linking the left subclavian artery to this vessel. The possible application of this to patients with congenitally narrowed segments of aorta, the so-called coarctation of the aorta, was considered by Blalock but he did not think that the human body would tolerate clamping the aorta for a sufficient length of time to carry out the anastomosis as it would entail cutting off the blood supply to the brain for a considerable period. That this could be done without causing serious brain damage was shown accident-ally by Crafoord, the Professor of Thoracic Surgery at the Karolinska Institute in Stockholm, who in 1942, while operating on a patent ductus, because of technical difficulties had to clamp the aorta for twenty-eight minutes. The absence of neurological sequelae in this case encouraged him to consider operating on the aorta for the relief of coarctation, and in 1944 he successfully resected a stricture of the aorta and then joined the two ends of the vessel together. Meanwhile, independent experimental dog work by Gross and Hufnagel on the problems of operating on the aorta which had been continuing in America since 1939 enabled Gross successfully to operate on patients with coarctation shortly after Crafoord's first case, and later Gross contributed further to the subject when he introduced the use of grafts of aortic tissue to bridge the gap when long strictures had to be resected. In Britain the operation was pioneered by Price Thomas (later Sir Clement Price Thomas) surgeon to the Westminster and Brompton Hospitals in London. But the great technical difficulties associated with the operation during those early days discouraged its widespread use by others for some years.

When Blalock presented the results of his experimental work to the staff at Johns Hopkins, Helen Taussig, the Associate Professor in Paediatrics there who had a special interest in congenital heart disease, suggested to him that he might be able to develop a method for increasing the flow of blood to the lungs in children with pulmonary valve stenosis by linking one of the main arteries arising from the aorta to the pulmonary artery. This led him to conduct further animal laboratory studies after which he invited Dr Taussig to send him some patients. The outcome of this was that the first 'blue baby' operation was performed on a child with the tetralogy of Fallot in 1944. The report of this, together with an account of the operation performed on two other children, was published by Blalock and Taussig in the *Journal of the American Medical Association* in 1945. Its dramatic nature immediately led to the greatest excitement and interest everywhere. Although the operation was not a direct attack on the anatomical defects present in this condition but a partial correction of them by the creation of yet another abnormality, it nevertheless brought considerable benefit to a large number of crippled children, firmly established cardiac surgery as a speciality in its own right, and paved the way for the development of more definitive methods of correcting valve deformities and septal defects. It was obvious that instead of by-passing the stenosed pulmonary artery it would be preferable to remove the obstruction. This was first achieved by Holmes Sellors (later Sir Thomas Holmes Sellors) surgeon to the Middlesex, National Heart, London Chest and Harefield Hospitals, who on 4 December 1947, when operating on a man with the tetralogy of Fallot and finding the Blalock type of by-pass operation technically impossible, thrust a long knife through the wall of the right ventricle and skilfully guided it by indirect palpation outside the heart until it reached the valve which he incised in two directions with marked improvement of the patient. Russell Brock (later Lord Brock), surgeon to Guy's Hospital and the Brompton Hospital, independently carried out a similar operation with success two months later, without either knowing of the other's work.

These blind procedures on the pulmonary valve performed on the unopened heart coincided with a revival of interest in operations for the relief of the far more common stenosis of the mitral valve. At first it was thought that the Cutler type of operation with incision into the valve cusps would be required but it soon became obvious that this was undesirable, and that it was better to stretch the orifice as had originally been done by Souttar. The first attempt was in 1945 when Charles Bailey, Professor of Thoracic Surgery at Hahnemann Medical School, in the United States, tried to cut out a piece of stenosed mitral valve but this was not successful. The next year he operated on another patient, planning to cut the valve by a knife passed through the left auricular appendage. During the operation the stenosis was found to be so severe that he could not do this so, remembering Souttar's original operation in 1925, he pushed his finger into the appendage and split the valve open with it. By 1948 Harken and Smithy, both in America, had successes with the use of dilating instruments, and in the same year Russell Brock in England carried out the Souttar-type operation of splitting the valve with his finger without at the time knowing anything of the work being done in the United States. This operation was so successful that he quite soon operated on seven more before publishing his results in 1950. Progress became so rapid that by 1952 Holmes Sellors was able to present a report to the European Congress of Cardiology of sixty-four of his own cases on whom he had operated without a single death. The operation was for some years performed by splitting the valve with the finger or occasionally by the use of special instruments passed through the left auricular appendage. In 1958 Logan and Turner in Edinburgh improved the results of the operation by passing a dilator through the wall of the left ventricle and guiding it through the mitral orifice with a finger placed in the left atrium.

The successful relief of stenosis of the pulmonary and mitral valves naturally led surgeons to attempt the same type of operation in cases of aortic stenosis but, unfortunately, the rock-like obstruction usually present in this disease, because of gross scarring and calcification of the valve, makes any blind dilating procedure extremely hazardous and gave disappointing results.

The stage had been reached where further progress in cardiac surgery required a technique whereby the heart could be excluded for a short time from the general circulation so that it could be opened and surgery performed under direct vision. This became possible when Bigelow, of Toronto, in 1952 cooled the body in order to reduce its oxygen and metabolic requirements sufficiently for the circulation to be arrested for a short period. He found that at a temperature of about 30° C the circulation could be stopped for a period of up to ten minutes. This now meant that not only was it possible to operate upon badly damaged valves but also that defects in the septum separating the atria and the ventricles could be repaired. The first success with open heart surgery occurred on 2 September 1952 when Lewis and his associates at the University of Minnesota Hospital, employing the technique of hypothermia at 30 °C closed an atrial septal defect. The methods of body cooling have varied, including lowering the temperature of arterial blood by passing it through a coil before returning it to the venous side of the circulation, but most popular of all has been surface cooling of the body by immersion in a bath of cold water. The obvious disadvantages of this technique was the limited period of time it gave the surgeons to operate, and although while sufficient for the suturing of a well-defined hole it was not long enough for more complex forms of repair. A further advance with the same technique was then made by Charles Drew, of the Westminster Hospital, who in 1959 developed and practised profound hypothermia with the body temperature reduced to 10–20°C which allowed cardiac arrest for forty to sixty minutes. The technique, although complex, has enabled many intricate procedures to be successfully completed.

The most widely used method however today, and one which allows the heart to be stopped for relatively long periods, is where the heart is by-passed and the blood pumped through an artificial oxygenator outside the body. The development of this technique was due to Gibbon, who became Professor of Surgery at the Jefferson Medical College in America. In 1931, after watching a patient at the Massachusetts General Hospital die from the effects of a massive blood clot impacted in the lung, he began to consider whether it would not be possible to keep such a patient alive until the clot had been surgically removed by having the work of the heart and lung performed artificially outside the body. With the assistance of his wife, Maly, he built a machine when at Harvard in 1934, capable of taking over the cardiorespiratory function of cats. As the years passed he improved the design of the apparatus, and in 1953 when he successfully repaired an atrial septal defect in an eighteen-year-old girl, he was the first surgeon to have operated on the open heart while the patient's blood was pumped through an extracorporeal oxygenator. She was connected with the apparatus for forty-five minutes, and for twenty-six minutes all cardiorespiratory function was taken over by the apparatus. In his report at the symposium on Recent Advances in Cardiovascular Physiology and Surgery at the University of Minnesota in September 1953 he said that the main feature of mechanical heart/lung apparatus is a suitable pump, his preference being for the De Bakey type of roller pump. And that the second important feature is the mechanical lung itself which in his machine allows oxygen to be absorbed and carbon dioxide released by spreading the patient's blood over both sides of screens with a mesh somewhat larger than that of fly screens whilst oxygen is blown over them. These screens are made of stainless steel wire suspended vertically and placed parallel in a plastic chamber.

Another approach to the problem was when Lillehei and his colleagues at the University of Minnesota oxygenated the blood of a patient undergoing open heart surgery by passing it through the circulation of another person. This crossed circulation technique was so dramatic that it attracted a great deal of public attention when first described in 1955, with newspapers and magazines reporting it widely. Many successful operations have been performed using this method but it is no longer used routinely. Improvements in the design of artificial heart/lung machines have continued with modified forms of Gibbon's original apparatus in use throughout the world today, enabling surgeons not only to repair complex septal defects but giving them the time required to complete complicated repair operations on valves and, more recently, to excise them and replace them either with valves from other people or from animals or by mechanical devices.

The wide choice of operation now available makes it essential for every patient with chronic heart disease to undergo an accurate assessment by a cardiologist with a detailed analysis of the history, skilful elicitation of physical signs, supplemented by information from X-rays and electrocardiographs. It is often possible, by these methods alone, to diagnose the type of structural damage and to assess the amount of disturbance of function in order to decide whether an operation would be helpful and if so what type would be best. In some cases, however, before such a decision can be made, it is essential for cardiologists to perform certain other rather more complex investigations for as one famous surgeon aptly said, 'a general going into battle wants to know whether he is going to meet a man on a bicycle or an armoured division, it is up to the cardiologist to tell us exactly what to expect'.

It was Werner Forssmann in Germany who first demonstrated that information could be obtained from direct instrumentation of the heart when, in 1929, having exposed a vein in his own arm, he inserted a catheter and advanced it into his right atrium. Initially, he developed the technique in order to get drugs quickly into the heart in an emergency to avoid the danger of injecting them by the blind insertion of a needle through the chest wall. He first practised on cadavers and found that he could thread a catheter through a vein in the front of the elbow into the right side of the heart. Courageously he then tried it on himself by persuading a colleague to insert a large needle into a vein in his arm through which he passed a catheter towards his heart. He stopped the experiment, however, because his friend thought it was dangerous. A week later, with boldness and determination, and completely alone, he anaesthetised the skin of his arm, incised the skin down to a vein and inserted a catheter in it for sixty-five centimetres, the distance he had estimated necessary to reach the heart. He then walked to the X-ray department and with the help of a nurse examined himself through a fluoroscope and confirmed that the catheter was in the right atrium. Next he used the method to inject drugs into the heart of a man very ill with a ruptured appendix. At the same time he predicted that the technique would be of value in studying the function of the heart, but it was not until 1941 that Cournand and Ranges in America developed a technique for this purpose. Its use in Britain was pioneered by John McMichael and E. P. Sharpey-Schafer of the British Postgraduate Medical School, London. It was with much courage that these men performed this investigation for the first time as many of those around them considered they would be submitting their patients to unjustifiable risks, so that they well knew, therefore, that if anything untoward should happen they would be subjected to the most stringent criticism. The immediate success of their method quickly silenced their critics and before long it became an established diagnostic procedure in all cardiological units. It is not performed as a routine preoperative procedure but reserved for selected cases such as when the anatomical diagnosis is uncertain as in complex congenital disorders with multiple anomalies; also for the accurate assessment of disturbance of function as well as to assist in the exclusion of factors which might preclude surgery.

The most commonly used catheter is known by Cournand's name and has a woven dacron base with a radio-opaque elastic compound applied over it. The instrument is guided into the heart under visual control using an image intensifier with a television monitor. A large number of skilled persons as well as expensive electrical and radiographic equipment are required. The catheter is readily passed through a vein into the right atrium, right ventricle and pulmonary artery but also may be manipulated through the septum from the right atrium into the left atrium. The left ventricle may be reached by introducing a catheter into an artery and passing it upwards against the stream of blood or alternatively by passing a needle through the skin directly into it. With an intracardiac catheter information may be obtained by observing whether it takes a normal path, by measuring the pressure gradient across valves as well as by estimating the oxygen content of blood in the various chambers. Also it is used in the performance of angiocardiography which involves the injection of an iodine-containing contrast medium into the circulation so as to

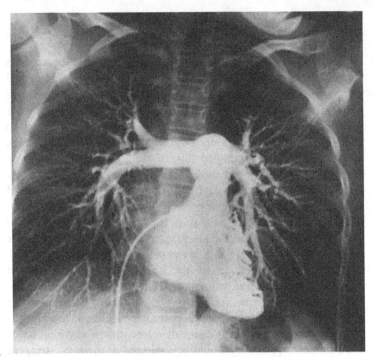

a

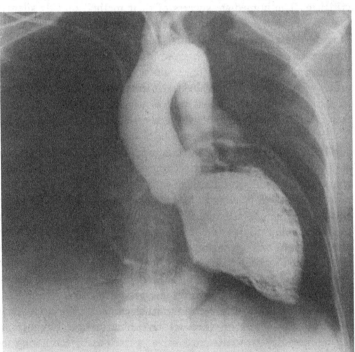

b

Angiocardiograms: (a) *shows radio-opaque dye filling the normal right ventricle and branches of the pulmonary artery;* (b) *shows dye filling a normal left ventricle and aorta and outlining the coronary arteries arising from the first part of the aorta* make the heart chambers, vessels and any abnormal communications radio-opaque. The material is injected very rapidly through the catheter into various selected sites in the heart and serial single pictures in rapid succession (six films per second) are then taken in two planes simultaneously or ciné-angiography is performed at thirty to sixty frames a second on thirty-five millimetre film. Serial films show structural changes to best advantage whilst disturbances of function and the direction of blood flow are best demonstrated by ciné-photography. For example, anatomical abnormalities such as a patent ductus or coarctation of the aorta are best seen on serial films whereas a jet of blood regurgitating through an incompetent valve is most clearly visualised on ciné film. Demonstration of the latter is, for example, often of vital importance in assessing the type of operation required for mitral valve disease as from the appearance of the jet the degree of reflux may be judged and this can often be of much help in deciding whether the valve is so irreparably damaged as to require replacement. Appreciable regurgitation of blood through the mitral valve always necessitates open heart surgery but the type of operation depends on the extent of the damage. When the regurgitation is due to destruction of tissue by bacterial endocarditis, or rupture of the chordae tendinae tethering the cusp edges, it is usually sufficient to repair the damage by plication of the cusps, or by plastic repair with addition of pericardial patches to deficient parts of the structure. Rheumatic disease, however, usually causes such extensive damage that replacement of the entire valve mechanism is required. Artificial valves of many types have been used but the one most widely employed is the one designed by Albert Starr, Professor of Surgery at the University of Oregon in America. This consists of a metal cage supporting a ball which moves freely up and down during systole and diastole. This gives excellent results but thrombosis around the valve and the resultant discharge of emboli into the circulation has meant that every patient has to have treatment with anticoagulant drugs. The incidence of this complication has been dramatically reduced since all the metal of the valve has been covered with a plastic velour cloth. Another approach has been to avoid metal cages altogether by replacing destroyed mitral valves by grafts of human or animal valves. Unfortunately, as there are technical difficulties associated with the use of transplanted mitral valves attempts have been made to insert aortic valves turned upside down into the mitral area. Unfortunately, grafts obtained from people who have died in accidents are always smaller than the dilated mitral valve rings into which they are to be inserted but Wooler and his colleagues in Leeds have shown that this problem may be avoided by the use of heterograft aortic valves from pigs and calves.

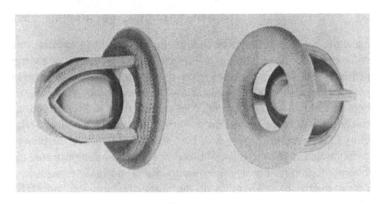

Starr Edwards artificial mitral valve

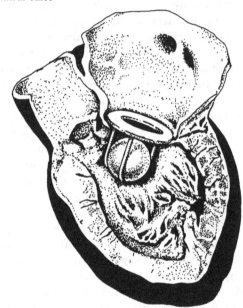

Starr Edwards valve replacing a damaged mitral valve

The removal of a damaged aortic valve and its replacement by one from a dead person was first carried out by Donald Ross in 1962 at the National Heart Hospital in London. Since then the procedure has been repeated many times in various parts of the world and proved to be highly successful. Valve transplants not only avoid the hazards of embolisation but being of perfect design allow unimpeded outflow of blood, in contrast to the central obstruction of mechanical prostheses.

The procedures so far described have now become the routine practice of every cardiac surgeon. There are other operations however which are for the most part still in the experimental stage

THE TRIUMPHS OF SURGERY 179

including surgery for coronary artery disease and heart transplantation. Efforts to ameliorate the effects of occlusion of the coronary arteries by surgery have included operations on the thyroid gland and the sympathetic nervous system both of which control the action of the heart; also procedures to augment the blood flow to the heart muscle as well as attempts to re-canalise blocked coronary vessels.

The metabolism of the body, including that of the heart, is under the control of the thyroid gland, and it will be remembered that Caleb Parry in 1825 drew attention to the increased rate of the heart when the thyroid gland is overactive. As angina occurs when the heart beats rapidly in response to exercise or emotion it is logical to attempt to control the heart rate. It was for this purpose that in 1933 Blumgart and his colleagues in America removed the thyroid gland in patients with intractable angina with favourable results. Thyroid gland activity can now be more readily controlled in patients over the age of forty by the administration of radio-active iodine, but thyroid suppression for angina is not widely practised at the moment as its place in the treatment of the condition has still not been clearly defined. The same rationale underlies the operation of sympathectomy whereby the sympathetic nerves to the heart are divided as it is the impulses from these nerves which cause the heart to beat faster and with increased force. This operation too has been superseded in recent years by the use of drugs, including propranalol, which block the nerve pathways by a chemical action. At one time it was considered unwise to abolish anginal pain as it removed a danger signal, but further experience has disproved this.

The surgeon who has devoted most interest to augmenting the blood flow to the heart muscle over the longest period of time is Claude Beck, Professor of Cardiovascular Surgery at Western Reserve University, who at least five years before the Second World War was insufflating asbestos talc around the heart muscle in order to produce an inflammatory reaction which would improve the blood flow, an operation which has been used with success from time to time. Also, he was the first to re-route blood from other parts of the body when about the same time he sutured a flap of muscle from the chest wall to the heart's surface. O'Shaughnessy, the promising young London surgeon, tragically killed during the evacuation from Dunkirk, used the same principle when in 1937 he sutured the omentum, the apron of tissue overlying the intestines, to the heart.

Vineberg in Canada improved upon this principle when in 1946 he mobilised the internal mammary artery and implanted its free end into a two-inch tunnel in the heart muscle so as to allow blood to seep into the sponge-like sinusoidal spaces which are in direct communication with the main coronary arterial system. This operation was at first received with scepticism as it was considered that the blood, instead of flowing freely, would coalesce into a large bruise or haematoma, but others have used it with great success, including the American, Effler, who by 1965 had treated seventy-six patients in this way.

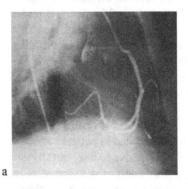 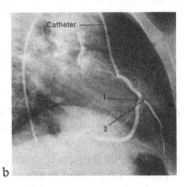

(a) *Coronary arteriogram—showing normal right coronary artery.* (b) *Coronary arteriogram—showing severe narrowing of the artery from atheromatous thickening of the wall at two sites (1 and 2)*

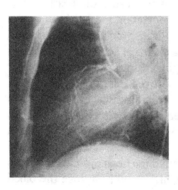

Coronary arteriogram—showing multiple small vessels normally closed but which have opened to provide a collateral circulation when the flow of blood through the main artery has become blocked

Recently, Mason Sones in America developed a method whereby the flow of radio-opaque dyes through the coronary arteries may be visualised by ciné-radiography. A very useful diagnostic procedure in certain atypical cases of chest pain where there is doubt as to whether or not the symptom is due to occlusion of the coronary vessels but also of use in the selection of cases where the disease is limited to involvement of one major vessel by a localised thrombus which might be removed. This however is a hazardous procedure and one which requires much improvement in technique before it can be employed routinely.

A large number of patients, as a result of rheumatic fever, or more commonly now, coronary artery disease, have such extensively damaged heart muscle that no treatment is of any avail other than heart transplantation. Public interest in this subject was particularly aroused when Professor C. Barnard and his team at the Groote-Schur Hospital, Cape Town, transplanted a heart from a twenty-five-year-old woman, mortally injured in a road accident, into fifty-five-year-old Louis Waskansky on 3 December 1967. This was rightly acclaimed as a magnificent achievement, although its performance immediately gave rise to questions of the highest ethical importance, and the death of Waskansky eighteen days after the operation highlighted the difficulties that surround such a feat in spite of the performance of skilled surgery. The operation had been preceded by much pioneer work over several years in many parts of the world. The technique of transplantation of organs had first been developed in experimental animals and application of this had already led to long-term successes with human kidney transplants. It was soon recognised that organs could be transferred without difficulty from one identical twin to another but that attempts to do this in other people led to the rejection of the foreign protein by the recipient. This resulted in a search for methods of matching tissues, similar to those developed for distinguishing blood groups by Landsteiner, over half a century ago. During the past three years it has become possible to identify antigens in the white cells of one individual which are compatible with those of another and this grouping of white cells into various types has been of some use in selecting suitable donors for kidney transplants. Although a certain degree of correlation has been found between tissue acceptance and white cell typing there have been many individual exceptions, with some renal grafts doing well, despite a major mismatch, but others doing badly in spite of apparent compatibility. This implies that this present method of tissue identification is of limited value and, although a distinct advance, is not the final solution.

Destruction of an implanted organ is brought about by the recipient's development of antibodies. The formation of these may be suppressed by irradiation of the tissues and the use of certain other agents including corticosteroids and azathioprine and anti-lymphocyte serum but at the cost of interfering with the other immunological processes in the body so that the patient's susceptibility to infection is markedly increased. Advances in the use of artificial kidney machines have improved the results of renal transplants in recent years because their employment for some time before operation allows renal failure to be successfully combated and is also of great use in supporting life during rejection crises. Unfortunately, there is no similar machine available to take the place of the heart so that accurate matching of the tissues of the donor and recipient is much more crucial and the operation will always have to be done on a patient whose health is seriously undermined by protracted and unrelieved cardiac failure.

The type of donor suitable for cardiac transplantation is a young adult with a healthy heart but whose brain has been severely damaged. The brain is not only the centre of the intellect but controls all the other functions of the body so that once irreparable brain damage has been sustained life cannot be maintained and the patient is in reality dead although the tissues of the body can be preserved for a time by mechanical devices. The very difficult decision therefore that has to be made in the case of a severe head injury in an otherwise suitable young person is whether or not the cerebral damage is irreversible. Relatives are then faced with the strain of deciding whether to give permission for the heart to be transplanted at a time when they are already subjected to considerable distress. The operation on the recipient in preparation for removal of the damaged heart must then first be started as it is impossible to keep the donor's heart viable for any length of time once removed from the body. This calls for the most careful co-ordination between two surgical teams and it is therefore instructive to study the timing of events during the first human heart transplant. The young woman, knocked over by a car shortly before 4 p.m. was admitted to hospital severely injured and deeply unconscious. Resuscitation was begun by a specially trained multiple injury service but by 9 p.m. her recovery seemed unlikely, and at 10 p.m. her breathing had to be assisted by a mechanical respirator. The patient was seen by an experienced neurosurgeon who considered her brain damage to be lethal and beyond treatment so that a decision was then made to use her heart to replace that of Waskansky, a diabetic who had suffered attacks of coronary thrombosis in 1959, 1960 and 1965 and who, since August 1967 had been in intractable heart failure. At 00.45 the donor was taken to the operating-theatre and artificial ventilation continued. At 00.50 the recipient was taken to another theatre and anaesthetised and at 1.30 the operation to remove his damaged heart was begun. At 2.20 artificial ventilation of the donor was discontinued and twelve minutes later her heart stopped, at which stage the operation to remove it was begun. The removed heart was ready for insertion into the recipient at 3 a.m. and was successfully implanted by 6.13 a.m. The battle to prevent the development of destructive antibodies then began with the use of drugs and irradiation of the heart from a cobalt bomb. It was not long however before evidence of commencing rejection necessitated an increase in the dose of drugs and the patient had to be nursed in isolation with strict aseptic precautions to avoid the introduction of infection. In spite of these measures the patient succumbed to a severe pneumonia.

Since then many other transplants have been done, including one by the same team in South Africa, on 2 January 1968, into a dental surgeon, Philip Blaiberg, which proved to be particularly successful; one by Donald Ross, Donald Longmore and Keith Ross, at the National Heart Hospital in London, on 3 May 1968; and several in America, most of them by Denton Cooley in Houston, Texas, many of whose patients temporarily returned to work. Some authorities consider that far greater accuracy in the matching of tissues and improved methods to combat tissue rejection are essential before cardiac transplantation can take its place as a routine procedure. When that day arrives other problems will arise including finding sufficient suitable donors for the very large number dying from degenerative heart disease. There is the possibility that this difficulty may be avoided by the invention of a mechanical heart or by the use of animals hearts, as, in fact, was done in 1964 when Hardy and his American colleagues transplanted a chimpanzee's heart into a man, although unfortunately in this case it only functioned for a few hours. Advances in human heart transplantation will undoubtedly proceed but, in the meantime, important problems in the care of the recipient remain to be solved and the signs of irreversible brain damage need to be carefully defined so that there can never be any doubt as to when death has occurred in a potential donor.

Surgery of the heart requires the combined efforts of a large team, it would be invidious to pick out for special mention any of the large number of contemporary physicians and cardiologists throughout the world who, by their diagnostic abilities and wise selection of cases, have done so much to advance this subject. Special reference, however, must be made to Paul Wood who was not only a superb physician but also a skilled physiologist and because of this was able to integrate knowledge gained by complex scientific apparatus with observations made at the bedside. His driving personality led him to demand high standards both from himself and those around him; he had a logical incisive mind and expressed his opinions fearlessly. His outspoken intolerance of slipshod thinking or ill-conceived ideas could on occasion cause offence. No one however doubted his complete sincerity or outstanding abilities. His gifts as a scientist, physician and teacher, were matched by those as a writer. His book *Diseases of the Heart and Circulation* was an analysis of his own vast clinical experience. He started to write it during the Second World War but lost the original manuscript in Italy whilst serving there with the army. It was eventually published in 1950 when it was immediately acclaimed as a masterpiece. During the years as a teacher at the Brompton and National Heart Hospitals in London after the war he had a profound influence on cardiological thought and practice so that his sudden death from coronary thrombosis in 1962 while still only in middle life was a grievous loss to world medicine.

The development of cardiac surgery has been one of the most outstanding achievements of the twentieth century. Dramatic and life-saving though it is, and whilst admiring the ingenuity of scientists and the supreme courage and skill of surgeons which have made it possible, its success must not be allowed to detract from the important, though less spectacular, progress made in the diagnosis, medical treatment and prevention of heart disease during the last fifty years. The prevention of rheumatic fever by the prompt control of streptococcal infections of the throat, and the avoidance of damage to the heart by the early and effective treatment of syphilis, both as a result of the discovery of penicillin, are measures which have greatly reduced the number of cardiac cripples. There will be another major advance when it is discovered how to prevent the development of atheromatous degeneration in the walls of vessels and thrombosis of the blood flowing through them. This will have a remarkable effect in increasing the life-span of individuals but at the same time, by increasing the proportion of old people in the community, will in its turn create its own social problems. Therefore, there remains much still to be done and in the words of Seneca, written nineteen hundred years ago: 'The opportunity of adding something will not be denied to anyone born a thousand ages later.'

Index of Persons

Subject Index